User Involvement in Health Care

User Involvement in Health Care

Edited by

Trisha Greenhalgh, OBE, MA, MD, FRCP, FRCGP
Professor of Primary Health Care and Director, Healthcare,
Innovation and Policy Unit Centre for Health Sciences
Barts and The London School of Medicine and Dentistry
London, UK

Charlotte Humphrey, PhD
Professor of Health Care Evaluation
King's College London
London, UK

Fran Woodard, MBA, DProf
Director, Cancer Programme
Integrated Cancer Centre
King's Health Partners
London, UK

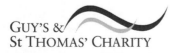

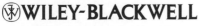

A John Wiley & Sons, Ltd., Publication

This edition first published 2011, © 2011 by Blackwell Publishing Ltd

BMJ Books is an imprint of BMJ Publishing Group Limited, used under licence by Blackwell Publishing which was acquired by John Wiley & Sons in February 2007. Blackwell's publishing programme has been merged with Wiley's global Scientific, Technical and Medical business to form Wiley-Blackwell.

Registered office: John Wiley & Sons Ltd, The Atrium, Southern Gate, Chichester, West Sussex, PO19 8SQ, UK

Editorial offices: 9600 Garsington Road, Oxford, OX4 2DQ, UK
The Atrium, Southern Gate, Chichester, West Sussex, PO19 8SQ, UK
111 River Street, Hoboken, NJ 07030-5774, USA

For details of our global editorial offices, for customer services and for information about how to apply for permission to reuse the copyright material in this book please see our website at www.wiley.com/wiley-blackwell

Library of Congress Cataloging-in-Publication Data
User involvement in health care / edited by Trisha Greenhalgh, Charlotte Humphrey, Fran Woodard.
    p. ; cm.
    Includes bibliographical references and index.
    ISBN 978-1-4051-9149-4
1. Patient participation–Great Britain.   2. Great Britain. National Health Service.
3. National health services–Great Britain.   I. Greenhalgh, Trisha.   II. Humphrey, Charlotte.   III. Woodard, Fran.
    [DNLM: 1. Great Britain. National Health Service.   2. Patient Participation–Great Britain.   3. State Medicine–Great Britain.   W 85 U84 2011]
    R727.42.U84 2011
    610.69′6–dc22

                                                                        2010024522

ISBN: 9781405191494

A catalogue record for this book is available from the British Library.

This book is published in the following electronic formats: ePDF 9781444325171; Wiley Online Library 9781444325164

Set in 9.25/12 pt Meridien by Aptara® Inc., New Delhi, India
Printed and bound in Singapore by Fabulous Printers Pte Ltd

1   2011

Contents

Contributors

Ceri Butler
Lecturer in Health Services Research
Division of Medical Education
University College London
UCL Medical School
London, UK

Paula Baraitser
Medical Adviser, English National Chlamydia Screening
  Programme
Consultant in Sexual Health
King's College Hospital NHS Foundation Trust
London, UK

Lizzy Bovill
Assistant Director of Operations
London Ambulance Service NHS Trust
London, UK

David Freedman
Freelance writer, London, UK

Trisha Greenhalgh
Professor of Primary Health Care
Queen Mary
University of London
London, UK

Jane Hughes
Research Fellow
Department of Interdisciplinary Studies in Professional Practice
School of Community and Health Sciences
City University London
London, UK

Charlotte Humphrey
Professor of Health Care Evaluation
King's College London
London, UK

Vikki Pearce
Programme Manager
NHS Tower Hamlets
London, UK

Gaynor Smith
End of Life Care Programme
Modernisation Initiative
St. Thomas' Hospital
London, UK

Fran Woodard
Director, Cancer Programme
Integrated Cancer Centre
King's Health Partners
London, UK

Foreword

This book draws on the collective experience of one of the largest, most visionary and most successful system-wide change initiatives in recent NHS history, that of the Modernisation Initiative of the Guy's and St Thomas' Charity.[1] The remit was to make a 'big difference' to local services by ensuring that the patient voice was the lifeblood of the programme.

Over a 3-year period, this initiative established a genuine partnership at all levels between service improvement experts, dozens of clinicians and over 500 patients and carers. This partnership proved a key catalyst in transforming the quality of care in local kidney, stroke and sexual health services.

When I was first asked to chair the Kidney Disease Modernisation Initiative (KDMI), I was absolutely stunned. I was at a loss for words. As a kidney patient for 25 years, this was the first time anyone had ever asked me – a patient – to contribute in any way to share my experience, improve services and help others.

Unsure whether to accept, I turned to a relative who exclaimed 'you must'! Surprised, I asked why. Recalling the recent D-Day commemoration, she explained, 'a soldier approached the lectern, but before he got there, before he even spoke, you absolutely knew that he had been there on that fateful day in 1944'. Pausing, she said 'Well, you are like that soldier, you yourself have really been there'! Though astonished, I took her advice. However, I still wasn't really sure how the patient experience could inspire change.

Then on a trip with clinicians to Holland it clicked. I finally understood. I got it! Chatting with other patients, I heard firsthand that 10 patients were so well, on a new nocturnal form of dialysis, that they no longer wanted a transplant! When you have hung on by the tips of your fingernails for 25 years to get a working transplant and have had 3 failed attempts already, your ears prick up when you hear this. It makes you sit bolt upright in your chair!

---

[1] This was actually the first of several Modernisation Initiatives funded by the Charity. For more details of the Charity's work see http://www.gsttcharity.org.uk/

What was going on? How could any dialysis patient *not want a transplant*? The answer appeared to be that this new treatment had led to an unprecedented improvement in their quality of life. Returning to England I gave a speech on behalf of the KDMI, advocating the adoption locally of nocturnal dialysis. Nearly a year later and after the incredible hard work of many clinicians and modernisers, the first patient in the United Kingdom to switch from standard to nocturnal dialysis, exclaimed with delight, 'I have just had my first pint of beer in 12 years'!... That long-awaited pint of beer wasn't on the evidence-based guidelines for managing kidney disease (which were, of course, important too) – but it did poignantly symbolise the difference the new service made to the patient experience.

It was only through the widespread and multi-level incorporation of patient experiences such as this that the Modernisation Initiative was able to achieve so much. Indeed there was such commitment to this vision and such integrity within the MI's leadership – especially the programme director, the managers and clinical champions – that no project was given the go ahead without some form of genuine patient and service user involvement.

If you have ever been touched or inspired by the experience of a patient or carer, and wished that you could translate that understanding and insight into improvements in services so as to make them more personalised and centred around individual patient needs, then this is the book for you.

If you have a vision of how care for a specific group of patients should be provided and want to work collaboratively with care providers to deliver new types of care, then this is the book for you.

If you have ever wanted to take the next step in patient engagement, to develop an ethos and governance structure in your organisation that encourages patients to emerge as teachers, early adopters and champions of change, then this is the book for you.

This book explains the techniques used by all three MI teams (stroke, kidney and sexual health) to help clinicians genuinely partner with patients and carers. It is also packed with practical tips and guidance on tools you can use to overcome many of the common challenges and pitfalls of delivering whole system change.

A few of the many tools covered in this book include: the use of mystery shoppers or whole system events to co-design new services, new units or new clinics; empowering patients to train staff in what 'good practice' means; the co-production of innovative information for patients and carers; and also the development of leadership roles for service users.

So what type of outcomes can be delivered when you systematically use these tools? Some of the changes the KDMI introduced, for example, included: new treatment options such as unit-based self-care and nocturnal dialysis that helped patients regain some control over their lives and improve their quality of life, innovative DVDs that enabled patients to make informed treatment choices that suited their lifestyle, peer to peer support that offered patients hope and helped them make the right decisions at the right time for them and a new palliative care option that supported patients to die where they wished.

So what did kidney care feel like after the modernisation process itself? Interestingly, for some patients, it was not just the new choices that mattered, it was also the change in the culture of the staff. According to one patient, 'The results of the MI were changes on the ward that made patients more comfortable, more empowered. Attitudes to patients have really changed. For example, now it is a 'let's do it together' attitude. For example, when taking blood, clinicians will now ask 'Where shall we put the needle'? There is a greater willingness to consult you, the person with the disease'.

My hope is that this book will inspire you with the confidence to take patient involvement to the next level in your areas. Delivering a service that is truly patient-centred is an enormous challenge, which can only be overcome by moving beyond a 'tick box' approach and actively engaging patients as a valuable resource.

I also hope that this book will help trigger a greater recognition of the value of the patient insight or experience. After all, it is patients who experience firsthand the chinks and cracks in the services. They often see and feel best practice in action and are the first to notice when it is not. As the quote from the patient above shows, these can be small things as well as large, system-wide changes. It is the patient rather than staff who will notice, for example, when a nurse take care to spray a local anaesthetic over deeply embedded stitches prior to removal to help reduce the pain, or conversely when someone is writhing in agony waiting for pain relief. It is the unparalleled authenticity of patient experience that presents ideas and opportunities for change.

By drawing on the rich and varied examples contained in this book, including the Top Ten Tips within in each section, I am confident that you will find, as we did, that partnering with patients in redesigning services is the most powerful way to deliver care that you know is centred on and actually meets individual needs. Importantly, involving patients may improve the morale and experience of staff. As one clinician explained, 'Involving patients is liberating, it empowers me...because I now know...that I focus on patient needs rather than what I think they need'. And in the words of another clinician, '[involving patients] has made me excited. Happier in my job...because the way that I am doing things is more meaningful, more directed by patients, more impactful'.

But it is not just clinicians who are excited about being involved, as one patient highlighted, '[Involvement] gave me a feeling of self-worth. It made me want to get out of bed each day. It is the only way that I can help other people'.

On a more personal note, empowering me to help make a difference in patient care has helped transform decades of inconceivable suffering, endless days and nights of hospitalisation, dialysis, operations and multiple transplantation, into what I now recognise is a gift. A gift to help others.

Jonathon Hope – Chair of the *Kidney Disease Modernisation Initiative*, May 2010

Acknowledgements

The Modernisation Initiative (MI) programmes described in this book and the independent evaluation of these were funded by a donation from the Guy's and St Thomas' Charity. As set out in this book, the programmes' success depended not only on the hard work and vision of numerous paid staff but also on the creative, tenacious and usually unpaid input of service users. We are grateful to the staff of the MI, clinical champions, service users and NHS staff involved in the projects, stakeholders in the four NHS Trusts, and trustees and officers of the Charity and others who contributed to the work of the various projects and the independent evaluation. We thank Mrs B J Garraway for kind permission to reproduce the picture of the late Mr Frederick Garraway on Page 57. The views expressed in this report are those of the authors and do not necessarily reflect those of the MI staff, its partner Trusts, the Charity or the academic institutions involved.

CHAPTER 1

User involvement – a story of our time

Trisha Greenhalgh[1], *Charlotte Humphrey*[2] *& Fran Woodard*[3]
[1]Queen Mary, University of London, London, UK
[2]King's College London, London, UK
[3]Integrated Cancer Centre, King's Health Partners, London, UK

Introduction

There is motherhood, there is apple pie and there is 'user involvement' in health care. Patients, carers, parents and advocates of the sick and vulnerable should have input into the kind of health service we have. They should be consulted about changes to services, and they should be involved in the design of those services. They should help to set the standards by which services are judged, and help to assess whether a particular aspect of the service meets those standards. At every stage, the users of the health service should be offered the opportunity to play an active part in developing, delivering and evaluating *their* service. After all, it is their (i.e. our) taxes which pay for it and their (our) lives which are at stake if things go wrong.

That all of this is taken as given is a measure of how far we have come since the bad days when health services were (many would say) designed for the convenience of doctors, nurses or managers. Patients in hospital had to lie in their beds waiting politely for the 'bedpan round', and their loved ones were banished at the end of the visiting hour by a shrill, uncompromising bell. People in pain from arthritis or a hernia waited months or years for a hospital outpatient appointment, and then went onto another waiting

---

list for their operation. General practitioners would shut up shop on the afternoons they played golf. If a chief executive wanted to axe the physiotherapy service, he or she did just that. The 'patient journey' (such as it was) was modelled on the Fordist principle of standardised, basic care with no frills and no choice. Few people complained – it was just the way things were.

Was it ever this bad? Probably not, but it is certainly true that over the past 15 years, there has been a sea change in what we in the UK expect of our National Health Service (NHS), and this has mirrored a wider change in expectations for health services across the western world. The first policy document to set out the vision for a transformed, patient-oriented health service in the UK was probably The NHS Plan in 2000.[1] In 2001, David Fillingham, head of the NHS Modernisation Agency (an 'arms length' body funded by the government to help NHS organisations become more efficient and patient-centred) captured the mood of the moment:

> The NHS has embarked upon a decade of improvement. Over the next ten years the delivery of care will be transformed as The NHS Plan is implemented. Care will be designed around the needs of patients and their carers. Diagnosis and treatment that previously took weeks or months will be completed in days or even hours.
> www.modern.nhs.uk, accessed January 2004

The various work programmes underpinning the NHS Plan were described by change management guru Professor Don Berwick of the US Institute of Health Improvement as '. . . to my knowledge, the most ambitious concerted systematic improvement effort ever undertaken, anywhere, by any organisation of comparable size' (Don Berwick, personal communication, July 2004).

And even in those early days of the new millennium, when tension for change was high and the funding allocated for NHS services was rising year-on-year, nobody believed it would be easy. As Chapter 2 illustrates, the research literature suggests that efforts to involve health service users in improving 'their' services have rarely gone entirely to plan.

This book is not a comprehensive guide to every possible approach to user involvement. Nor is it an account of unqualified success or a 'how-to' guide, which will allow you to replicate in any simple way the things that went well. It is a story of a single programme of work, involving hundreds of people, which happened in inner London in the mid-2000s. It was called the modernisation initiative (MI), and it began when several front-line teams were all lucky enough to share a generous donation of funding from a well-endowed local charity to 'modernise' health services on their patch.

The book describes how the different teams involved in the MI went about involving service users in deciding how the money should be spent and pushing through the changes that were deemed to be needed. And it tells the story of the patients, carers and other service users who came forward to make their contribution. The story of the MI, like all good stories, contains both successes and disappointments and a good many twists in the plot. But it is a real story, and despite not providing easy answers, it does offer useful insights for those embarking on similar challenges.

Most of the chapters in the book are written by the front-line staff and service users who worked on the MI. Three chapters – this introduction, the literature review in Chapter 2 and the discussion and conclusion in Chapter 8 – were written by members of the academic team who were contracted by the funders of the project to evaluate the work (Trish Greenhalgh, Charlotte Humphrey and Ceri Butler), with input from the person who was, at the time, the Director of the MI (Fran Woodard). We have published a full report on this programme elsewhere,[2] as well as some academic papers[3, 4] and internal reports on specific sub-projects.[5] The remainder of this chapter gives a summary of what the MI was and how it came about.

The modernisation initiative

The MI was a system-wide transformational change programme working across the health economy in the London boroughs of Lambeth and Southwark to modernise local health services. It was formed as a local partnership between Guy's and St Thomas' NHS Foundation Trust (GSTT), King's College Hospital NHS Foundation Trust (KCH), Lambeth Primary Care Trust, Southwark Health and Social Care Trust, community groups, patient groups and the independent and voluntary sector. The project was funded by a donation of £15 million from Guy's and St Thomas' Charity (the Charity).

The setting for the MI was Lambeth and Southwark, two adjacent inner London boroughs. This locality has all the challenges of a deprived inner city area – poverty, poor housing, high burden of disease, low health literacy, high population turnover, linguistic and ethnic diversity, numerous socially excluded groups and historically fragmented and uncoordinated services. Some individuals registered as patients with different parts of the service did not actually live in the area and, conversely, many residents who used services elsewhere, were not registered, or failed to access services at all.

In 2000, the large and long-established Guy's and St Thomas' Charity decided to invest a substantial sum of money for service transformation. This was something of a break in tradition. An informal local review in the late 1990s had revealed that although the Charity's funds were being drawn on in many ways by local health care projects, the impact of these various grants was unclear except in the case of major building projects. At that time there was growing recognition, more generally, that significant service change is rarely achieved through narrowly focused, short-term, small-scale projects. The idea was mooted among the Charity's trustees that major sustained investment in service transformation on a scale comparable to that required to build and equip a new hospital ward might well deliver better results. Fortuitously, a review of the Charity's accounts at about the same time identified some reserves that could be made available to be spent in a different way without reducing the amount of money already going to the type of projects it had traditionally funded.

Bids were invited from local services for three 'modernisation' projects, with the over-arching principle that the grants made would be large (£5 million per project) and should be used to make a 'big difference' to local services. It was expected that fundamental changes would be made in the way services were designed and delivered; the nature, quality and accessibility of services on offer; the attitudes of staff and (more broadly) the general culture of the services; the balance of power between patients and professionals; the way different parts of the health economy communicated and worked together; and – most significantly of all – the way in which patients, carers and communities were consulted and partnered in the planning and delivery of services.

The vision was thus for a more efficient, more integrated, more patient-focused service which reflected an NHS that was fit for the twenty-first century. The changes were expected to span both primary and secondary care (and, where appropriate, the voluntary and private sectors too) and to cover the entire patient pathway from prevention to end-of-life care. Whilst the pump-priming money was generous, the costs of the transformed service were expected to be met by the local health economy after the 3-year transformation period was over.

In early 2002, three projects – stroke services, kidney services and sexual health services – were identified in a competitive bidding process as potentially eligible for a grant of £5 million each. Once chosen, the three MI projects moved into an 'invention' phase – a 6-month period of 'energising, consultation, consensus building and discovering ideas' – aimed at refining the proposals, pulling together background information about services across all the partner organisations, identifying clinical champions, looking at ways to involve users, gathering innovative ideas, identifying areas of best practice elsewhere and arranging visits to them to learn more. Workshops were held with patients and voluntary organisations to develop the initiatives and outline applications were worked up for submission to the Charity. In November 2002, the Trustee Board approved funding for all three projects for a 1-year 'incubation' phase to work up implementation plans and consider how progress against goals would be assessed. The major tranche of funding was awarded to the stroke and kidney projects in late 2003, and 6 months later to the sexual health project.

The goals of the three MI projects are summarised in Box 1.1.

The management and governance of the MI was complex. An over-arching MI Board was established with representation from the four participating Trusts and other key stakeholders, and this met quarterly. Within each project, there was a management board which met approximately monthly and received reports from numerous sub-projects. Each project had a manager and lead clinician; the project managers were answerable to the MI Director, who had a clinical background (physiotherapy) but had worked for many years in various change management projects across the NHS. User representation on the different boards and management groups is discussed in Chapter 6.

In summary, the MI consisted of three linked projects, each of which was ambitious, multifaceted and oriented to transforming what was seen as an old-fashioned service in both primary and secondary care. They shared an over-arching vision (to make a 'big difference' to services locally and change them in a patient-centred way) and governance structure but their detailed goals and work plans were very different. Aside from being one of the largest and most challenging change projects ever undertaken in the UK health

Box 1.1 Goals of the three MI projects as set out in early business plans

Stroke
- Prevent people having strokes and encourage healthy lifestyles
- Ensure early detection of strokes
- Provide rapid access to early evidence-based interventions and treatments for all stroke patients
- Provide high quality, timely, consistent rapid access to rehabilitation within the community
- Facilitate people to have the best quality of life whilst living with the consequences of having a stroke (long-term support)

Kidney
- Prevent people developing kidney disease
- Increase the ability of primary care professionals to manage the early stages of kidney disease
- Reduce the waiting times in outpatient clinics and on dialysis units
- Improve the experience for patients staying on the wards
- Increase the treatment choices available to dialysis patients
- Increase the number of transplant operations by increasing the number of living donor operations
- Ensure appropriate supportive care is provided to patients when necessary
- Ensure appropriate services are provided to enable patients to 'live well' with kidney disease

Sexual health
- Reduce rates of sexually transmitted infections (STIs) and unintended pregnancy
- Reduce the number of people with undiagnosed asymptomatic STIs by increasing screening opportunities
- Increase opportunities for people to manage their own sexual health in supported environments
- Improve knowledge about sexual health and sexual health services especially in high-need communities

- Improve waiting times, staff attitudes and clinic environments
- Focus specialist resources on specialist need and developing additional capacity
- Establish a network that enables services to work together to consistent, evidence-based standards
- Improve the patient experience of using existing services by reducing waiting times

economy, the MI also offered a unique opportunity to learn lessons about how transformational change happens and how best to go about it.

An independent evaluation of the MI was commissioned by competitive tendering and the contract awarded to an interdisciplinary team of academics from University College London, King's College London, University of Surrey and University of Leeds. The evaluation was funded from August 2005 until July 2008 – somewhat later than the projects themselves. The Charity's requirements of the independent evaluation were that it should provide both formative feedback to support the implementation of the MI (hence, the evaluation team presented regularly to the MI Board and to a separate Evaluation Advisory Group) and summative feedback on the overall success of the programme (hence, we produced a lengthy final report to the Trustees). In addition, the evaluation team was asked to generate learning about the relationship between context, mechanism and outcome in service transformation and explore the implications for the funding of similar initiatives in the future.

The design of the evaluation took account of the fact that each of the three MI projects had many objectives and multiple work streams operating within and across the local health care system and community at a variety of levels, and that these different initiatives were likely to change organically with time. The approach taken was realist evaluation, which uses a variety of methods (mainly but not exclusively qualitative) to explore the interplay between context, mechanism and outcome.[6] In realist terminology, user involvement can be thought of as a 'mechanism' by which service transformation might be achieved, and this 'mechanism' will be more or less successful in different contexts. For those interested in academic aspects of how realist evaluation was applied to this programme of work, please see our published papers.[3,4]

Whilst this book can be read without a detailed knowledge of the academic aspect of realist evaluation, the key questions addressed by all the chapters, especially the analysis sections in Chapters 7 and 8, might usefully be expressed in the format used by Pawson and Tilley[6]: 'What works, for whom, in what circumstances when seeking to involve users in service transformation?' Furthermore, the very broad mechanism of 'user involvement' can be divided into a number of more specific sub-mechanisms – for example, working with service users to co-design services (see Chapter 3); using patients and carers as teachers to convey the illness experience and user priorities to staff and also to support other patients (see Chapter 4); co-producing information with service users (e.g. making leaflets or DVDs, see Chapter 5); or appointing service users to formal leadership and governance roles within a project (see Chapter 6). These sub-mechanisms might be employed in isolation or (perhaps better) synergistically with one another.

The next chapter completes this introductory section by offering a brief literature review on what is already known about user involvement in service transformation. The four subsequent chapters, which comprise the main section of the book, consider the four different sub-mechanisms for involving users and give examples from the different sub-projects in the MI of where these sub-mechanisms met with success, failure or partial success. The final section of the book synthesises the learning across all three projects and different approaches to user involvement by considering the various tensions and paradoxes which are inherent in attempts to involve users in service transformation (see Chapter 7) and offering some recommendations for future policy and research (see Chapter 8).

References

1. Department of Health. *The NHS Plan*. London: NHS Executive; 2000.
2. Greenhalgh T, Humphrey C, Hughes J, Macfarlane F, Butler C, Connell P et al. *The Modernisation Initiative Independent Evaluation: Final Report*. London: University College London; 2008.
3. Macfarlane F, Hughes J, Humphrey C, Pawson R, Butler C, Greenhalgh T. A new workforce in the making? A case study of strategic human resource management in a whole-system change effort in healthcare. *J Health Organ Manage* 2010; in press.

4. Greenhalgh T, Humphrey C, Hughes J, Macfarlane F, Butler C, Pawson R. How do you modernize a health service? A realist evaluation of whole-scale transformation in London. *Milbank Q* 2009; **87**(2):391–416.

5. Hughes J, Wood E, Cox S, Silas L, Smith G. 'No white coat between us'. *Developing Peer Support Services for Kidney Patients*. London: Modernisation Initiative; 2008. Available at http://www.gsttcharity.org.uk/pdfs/whitecoat.pdf.

6. Pawson R, Tilley N. *Realistic Evaluation*. London: Sage; 1997.

CHAPTER 2

What is already known about involving users in service transformation?

Ceri Butler[1] *& Trisha Greenhalgh*[2]
[1]Division of Medical Education, UCL Medical School, University College London, London, UK
[2]Queen Mary, University of London, London, UK

Introduction

The idea of involving 'users' in service transformation is not new. With its diverse origins in socialist political philosophy, consumerism, mental health activism and the 'survivor' movement, user involvement has more recently come to be seen as a key vehicle for the delivery of a more efficient, more integrated and more patient-focused health service for the twenty-first century.

In this chapter we explore the growing literature on user involvement. We have not attempted a complete review of the full range of literature on user involvement. Rather, we have sought to explore its conceptual foundations. We also take a brief look at the UK health sector's experience of user involvement and highlight where efforts to involve health service users in improving their services have not always gone to plan. We then move on to focus more specifically on the foundations for the 'whole systems' approach taken by the modernisation initiative (MI).

User Involvement in Health Care, 1st edition. Edited by Trisha Greenhalgh, Charlotte Humphrey and Fran Woodard. © 2011 Blackwell Publishing Ltd.

The UK experience

In the United Kingdom, user involvement in the health sector has a long history. It began formally with the creation of the Community Health Councils in 1974. These bodies sought to represent the interests of the public in the National Health Service (NHS). More recently, the renewed impetus for increasing patient and public involvement in the health sector has followed the introduction of the NHS internal market in the early 1990s and the transition from 'patients' to 'customers' or 'consumers' that was linked to this cultural shift in the health economy.[1]

The 1980s and 1990s saw a series of policy papers advocating a more 'consumerist' approach to health care. *The Griffiths Report* published in 1983 introduced the idea of producing 'satisfied customers' in the NHS.[2] The patient's role as customer or consumer was further set out in the legal statute *NHS and Community Care Act* 1990[3] and in *Local Voices: The Views of Local People in Purchasing for Health* in 1992.[4] Health authorities were advised to consult and involve voluntary agencies and user groups to draw up priorities and contracts for health and social care.

Another major impetus to the growing interest in user involvement in the NHS was the series of high-profile service failures such as that involving paediatric cardiac surgery in the Bristol Royal Infirmary,[5] the hundreds of murders committed by GP Harold Shipman,[6] and the failure to seek consent from parents for research use of organs of children who had died at Alder Hey hospital in Liverpool.[7] All these incidents were associated with extensive press coverage and major public inquiries, and a sea change in public trust in healthcare systems.[8] Partly as a result of these scandals, user involvement came to be seen as a central delivery vehicle for quality improvement, safety assurance and patient protection in health care.

Following the 1997 general election, the new Labour Government put forward 'even more eclectic influences that have encouraged participatory initiatives' and argued that a strategy of inclusiveness and consultation would achieve better policies and (hence) outcomes.[9] Two documents, *In the Public Interest: Developing a Strategy for Public Participation in the NHS*, published in 1998, and *Patient and Public Involvement in the New NHS*, published a year later, set out the Government's strategy to support public involvement in the NHS focusing on outcomes for the health service, its users, public health and local communities.[10, 11] The following list of benefits is taken from those documents:

Benefits to the NHS
• Restoration of public confidence
• Improved outcomes for individual patients
• More appropriate use of health services
• Potential for greater cost-effectiveness
• Contribution to problem resolution
• Sharing responsibilities for healthcare with the public

Benefits to people
• Better outcomes of treatment and care
• An enhanced sense of self-esteem and capacity to control their own lives
• A more satisfying experience of using health services
• More accessible, sensitive and responsive health services
• Improved health
• A greater sense of ownership of the NHS

Benefits to public health
• Reduction in health inequalities
• Improved health
• Greater sense of understanding of the links between health and the circumstances in which people live their lives
• More healthy environmental, economic and social policies

Benefits to communities and to society as a whole
• Improved social cohesion
• A healthy democracy – reducing the democratic deficit
• A health service better able to meet the needs of its citizens
• More attention to crosscutting policy issues and closer cooperation between agencies with a role to play in health improvement

Linking patient involvement with improving health outcomes was given increasing precedence in the early 2000s. Drawing on the pioneering work of Kate Lorig, a nurse who developed the Stanford model to support patients' involvement in their own care,[12, 13] the UK Government was determined to focus on an 'expert patient' programme as a way of managing the growing burden of chronic diseases.[14, 15] The white paper *Saving Lives: Our Healthier Nation* set out this commitment in 1999,[16] and the past 10 years have seen the introduction of a wide range of expert patient programmes in primary and secondary care. Such approaches are not without their critics, however. Radical academics have argued that 'expert patient' models are less about truly involving users and more about shifting responsibility for biomedical data collection and decision-making from the health system to the patient under a rhetoric of 'empowerment'.[17–19]

The white paper *The NHS Plan*, published in 2000, was the centrepiece of New Labour's modernising strategy for the NHS.[20] This document set out a series of targets for expanding the workforce, reducing waiting times and redesigning the health service around the needs and preferences of the patient. This ambitious vision for fundamental, transformational change across the whole of the NHS was followed up by an implementation plan.[21] A key element of this plan was the establishment of the NHS Modernisation Agency in 2001 with a remit to drive through reforms through improving access, increasing local support, raising standards of care and capturing and sharing knowledge across organisations.

With the renewed emphasis on improving public confidence in the health service and placing patient-centred care at the heart of modernisation,[11] the Health and Social Care Act 2001 placed a statutory duty on all NHS trusts, primary care trusts (PCTs) and strategic health authorities (SHAs) to involve and consult patients on the planning and provision of local services. A follow-on document, *Shifting the Balance of Power*, published in 2001, called for the introduction of a new patient advocacy and liaison service (PALS) and increases in the citizen and lay membership of professional regulatory bodies and the new NHS modernisation board.[22] Interestingly, when the PALS services were set up, the 'A' in the acronym had been mysteriously changed to 'Advice', with the effect that the advocacy element of these statutory bodies was downplayed.

Despite positive messages from central government and the Department of Health about user involvement in health services, some official initiatives were short lived. The Commission for Patient and Public Involvement in Health (CPPIH) was abolished only 18 months after being established in 2003, allegedly because of lack of grass roots support.[23] In the last few years, patients have been encouraged to become more involved in the their own health care through the introduction of personalised care plans and personally controlled budgets for those with long term conditions[24] and by the creation of the local involvement networks (LINks) as an additional voice for patients and service users in local areas. LINks were intended to promote and support the involvement of people in the commissioning, provision and scrutiny of local care services and to aid NHS providers to improve services through engagement with the local community.[25] The delay in actually establishing the LINks, however, attracted much criticism, with claims that 'public and patient involvement in health and social care has been seriously set back'.[26]

User involvement in governance (covered in Chapter 6) has a significant history within the NHS. For example, it operates at board level throughout the NHS, non-executive directors (NEDs) sit on the boards of all health trusts and SHAs. The National Institute for Health and Clinical Excellence (NICE) also includes lay people, patients and carers on its committees and working groups (http://www.nice.org.uk/getinvolved/). But whilst representation at board level is almost universal in the NHS, the actual power of users in such roles in UK public bodies has been questioned. In a study of nine projects in Wales involving citizens, for example, Adamson and Bromiley came to the following two key conclusions:

> *Participating community members feel empowered and have a positive 'can do' attitude about their ability to promote positive change in their community. However, the statutory sector has largely failed to respond to the community agenda and there is little evidence of community influence over budgets and service delivery, and no evidence of bending mainstream services to reflect the partnership process.* (p. xv)[27]

The rising interest at national policy level in user involvement should be seen as closely linked to the wider drive to improve healthcare quality while also reducing its cost. To some extent, user involvement is seen as a mechanism to achieve this 'better quality, lower cost' equation. This has similarly been the case in the United States with the Institute of Health Improvement (characterised by a highly technical, quantitative approach to measuring improvements).[28] However, despite the many developments that have taken place in the United Kingdom over the last 30 years, a survey from the UK-based Picker Institute claims that England remains behind Australia, Canada, New Zealand, Germany and the United States in public/user involvement.[29]

What is 'user' involvement and who are these 'users'?

Despite the numerous policy documents on involving service users there is no clear definition of user involvement.[30] How users are involved – or seen as potentially becoming involved – varies from one policy document and setting to another. In later chapters of this book, we will look in more detail at how service users were actually involved in the case of the MI but more generally, 'user involvement' may include any of the following (and probably other inputs too):

- Making decisions about their own health care
- Co-designing services,[31] redesigning services,[32] developing services[32] or change management[33]
- Teaching professionals and developing learning materials
- Undertaking peer education and support
- Capacity building[34]
- Staff recruitment[35]
- Clinical governance activities and/or the development of clinical guidelines[33]
- Evaluating service provision[36]
- Taking part in research[37, 38]
- Sitting on steering groups and other governance roles[39]

While there is substantial evidence of the impacts that user involvement can have on improved health outcomes in particular situations,[32] the wide-ranging methods of involvement make it impossible to make definitive, generalisable statements on the overall impact that 'user involvement' has across the health sector. There have been suggestions that randomised controlled trials would allow the impact of user involvement to be appropriately measured,[40] though this suggestion raises an interesting paradox – should researchers be entitled to randomise users like experimental animals to being 'involved' or not? Perhaps yes, but only if the users agree.

What you call individuals who 'use' health services is a topic of controversy. The UK Department of Health defines a service user as 'any person who has, is, or may access NHS or independent sector health services'.[11] But this definition has been challenged. Beresford, for example, sees the term 'service user' as presenting people in an essentially passive or consumerist way rather than as an active participant in decision-making.[41]

The terms 'users', 'survivors', 'clients', 'public', 'patients' and 'consumers' each bring different symbolic meanings and convey a different picture of what the transaction is about. In the mental health setting, Peck and Barker make a clear distinction between 'users' as consumers who want to participate more and 'survivors' who want to fundamentally change the foundations of the services themselves (both of which are perhaps different from 'patients' who simply wish to receive healthcare).[42]

Theoretical models of user involvement: choice and voice

There are numerous conceptual and theoretical models for considering the involvement of users in service change, and this chapter does not cover them all. In particular, some models of user involvement couch this process in terms of challenging social injustice, either as a social movement which criticises the status quo or more radically in overt conflict with the system and the state.[18, 43, 44] Such approaches are not covered here – not because we reject them but because the particular change initiative whose processes and mechanisms we were seeking to illuminate the modernisation initiative or MI couched user involvement in more conventional terms. Put bluntly, whilst user involvement was strongly supported by the MI, it would almost certainly have been seen as inappropriate for those charged with 'promoting user involvement' to encourage users to complain about the structure of society or the link between inequality and illness.

The two main conventional approaches to user involvement have been termed the 'democratic' and the 'consumerist' models. Below, we explore these two models and then discuss how the whole systems approach to user involvement draws partially but not fully on them. In this section, we are indebted to a review by Ian Greener who introduced the twin concepts of 'choice' and 'voice'.[45] He based his analysis on a 1970 article by Hirschman who suggested that 'individuals, wishing to improve the service they receive, have two main strategies: exit or voice'. By 'exit', Hirschman meant moving to another provider; by 'voice', he meant complaining or demanding improved services from their existing provider.

The democratic model (what Greener called 'voice'[45]) aims to enhance influence and control over the services we use. The idea of introducing democracy to a therapeutic community is not new and in the mental health setting dates back to the mid 1940s.[46] In modern day discussions we tend to link the democratic model dating back to the late 1960s with Arnstein's ladder of citizen participation. This model was originally developed in the context of urban redevelopment whereby participation was seen as a proxy for power.[47]

Arnstein's model has long been critiqued for its static, linear nature and for not considering the different types of, and contexts for, involvement. Such criticisms are well summarised by Tritter and McCallum in 2006:

> *A linear, hierarchical model of involvement – Arnstein's ladder – fails to capture the dynamic and evolutionary nature of user involvement. Nor does it recognise the agency of users who may seek different methods of involvement in relation to different issues and at different times. Similarly, Arnstein's model does not acknowledge the fact that some users may not wish to be involved.*[48]

Concerns about the inclusivity and representativeness of the user thus challenge this 'democratic' model. Arnstein's apparent assumption that all users would be somehow involved does not consider users who do not wish to be involved nor does it reflect the diversity of service users, the conditions they may seek care for or the circumstances in which they find themselves.

In recent years there has also been an increase in the number of 'professional' service users (individuals who began as 'ordinary' patients or carers but who gradually acquired specialist skills and knowledge, making them (allegedly) uniquely qualified to contribute to the development of services). However, much has been written about whether such 'professional' service users can represent the wider service user community precisely once they have become so familiar and comfortable with the healthcare system. As far back as the late 1970's Illich warned us of the dangers of the professionalisation of patients and trend of experts creating more experts.[49]

Linked to the formalisation (and perhaps professionalisation) of service users is the issue of payment. Should service users be paid for the time they devote to helping improve services? The UK Department of Health supports this principle but considers that the level of payment should depend on the level of commitment, individual skills and expertise.[50] We take up this theme in Chapter 7.

The context in which service users are involved is important in determining the likely impact that they will have. Institutional practices, hierarchical power structures and professional barriers play a significant role. A major review on user participation in social care by the Social Care Institute for Excellence in 2007 concluded that 'difficulties with power relations were found to underlie the majority of identified problems with effective user-led change. Exclusionary structures, institutional practices and professional attitudes can affect the extent to which service users can influence change'.[51]

In his 2006 critical realist review of user involvement in psychiatric services, Stickley concluded that after decades of user involvement, the powerful 'institution of psychiatry' continued to dominate. It was now time, he felt, that users stood up and challenged the prevailing hierarchy to effect real user-led change.[44] In other words, in situations where there is a large power differential, democratic models of user involvement were unlikely to succeed. This view was expressed back in 1971 by Edelman, who depicted democratic models of user involvement as 'symbolic acts' rather than as truly empowering users and capturing their views or needs.[52] Whilst not all scholars agree with this radical view, there is certainly a general perception that this model of user involvement may have inbuilt inequalities which are not always apparent to those who seek, in good faith, to use it in improving services.

It is worth briefly mentioning how this model of user involvement has fared in healthcare improvement initiatives outside the United Kingdom. In many younger democracies throughout the world, there is much sympathy with the idea of patient/user involvement, and initiatives with this generic aim continue to grow. But many of these are couched in the biomedical model of 'patient participants' which (arguably) reproduces the very power differentials between patients and professionals which it purports to challenge. South Africa, for example, has introduced a post apartheid policy of 'Batho Pele' ('People First'), with an explicit set of principles which all public bodies are expected to follow (http://www.nwdc.co.za/articles/Batho-Pele-Principles.pdf). This initiative is very much focused on 'get[ting] public servants to be service orientated, to strive for excellence in service delivery and to commit to continuous service delivery improvement'.[53] It is beyond the scope of this book to offer a detailed analysis of such initiatives and their critics, but it is worth commenting that the criticisms currently being directed at the well-intentioned Batho Pele policy parallel those that were directed at Arnstein's model in the United Kingdom a generation before.

The consumerist model (what Greener called 'choice'[45]) is not new but has become steadily more prominent in the past 40 years since Hirshman proposed his original 'exit' model. The growth in what has been called 'welfare consumerism' has been linked to the increase in average levels of income and a general rise in people's expectations of a long, healthy, symptom-free and risk-free life.[54] The public in general are demanding that 'public services become as responsive and dynamic as the private services they consume'.[45]

The basis of this model is 'economic man' [or woman] as a rational decision maker, who is able and willing to make choices between services and enact those choices. It assumes that in relation to healthcare, everyone knows what is best for them or has access to the information needed to find out. It also assumes that service users who intend to 'vote with their feet' have available a full range of options representing best quality care. Arguably, however, such situations are rarely the case in health care. Greener cites a study by Schwarz which showed that the vast majority of us, if asked before we got ill, 'would' like a choice of different providers if we were diagnosed with a serious illness, but that once someone has actually been diagnosed with a serious illness, only a small minority would still like a choice.[45] In such situations, most of us depend on, and defer to, the medical experts – and such things as trust, continuity of care and the therapeutic relationship become greater priorities than 'choice'.[55]

The strongest critics of the consumer model of user involvement are those who take issue with its political basis. John Clarke has referred to the 'subordination of social policy to the economy', and argued that by encouraging sick individuals to 'choose' their health care, the government is merely shifting responsibility from the well to the sick and from the state to the individual.[17] The terminology of the consumerist model has been vociferously challenged. Calling service users 'consumers' implies that a payment is made for services. In reality most 'consumers' receive free services in the public sector.[56] However, it is also true that the increased choices made available to NHS patients and the introduction of individual care budgets means that money does now to some extent follow the patient's choice of services.[57] Again, it is beyond the scope of this book to take sides on the issue of whether consumerism 'works' in user involvement but it is important to highlight that whilst some people view this as an important mechanism of change, others view it as wholly or partly symbolic and/or politically motivated.

Internationally, the consumerist model of user involvement is gaining popularity. Australia, for example, has an official policy of involving 'health consumers' in service improvement. The Consumers' Health Forum of Australia is a voluntary-sector organisation whose remit is 'representing and involving consumers in health policy' (see https://www.chf.org.au/index.asp).

Contemporary approaches to user involvement: co-design, co-production, co-leadership and mutual learning

As Chapter 1 explained, the whole systems approach to change goes beyond most local and national service improvement initiatives and seeks to achieve whole scale change in multiple different parts of the service and multiple different aspects of care. Whole systems change reflects the complexities and challenges of providing quality health care in the new health economies of the twenty-first century. Neither the democratic nor consumerist models of user involvement are sufficiently complex or nuanced to explain how users might contribute to such a multifaceted approach.

User involvement and participation in the modern era is characterised by:
- Accelerated rates of change – in medical knowledge, information systems and new technologies of treatment;
- Highly mobile and heterogeneous populations;
- Globalised health systems and service providers;
- Unprecedented complexity of local health economies, with multiple providers, funding systems and accountabilities;
- Uneven distribution of knowledge, wealth and influence which goes beyond a simple 'doctor has all the power, patient has none' equation;
- Diverse values and expectations among both service providers and recipients.

It follows, perhaps, that there is probably no one 'best way' to involve users, nor one 'best theory' to explain the success or failure of users in whole system transformation. As one document describing a whole systems change effort outside the healthcare sector put it:

> *Organisations must change at every level, from senior management to front line staff, if they want to achieve meaningful participation. [...] Participation should become part of daily practice, not a one-off activity. [...] Participation operates at different levels. There are many ways to involve service users in different types of decisions.*[57]

Successful user involvement in whole systems change efforts is thus likely to involve a wide variety of practical approaches *and* a range of different conceptual and theoretical models of who users are and how they might contribute to service improvement.

We believe that in today's complex, rapidly-changing (dare we say 'post-modern'?) world, we need to go beyond both 'left wing' models (which talk in terms of 'democratisation' and 'participation') and 'right wing' models (which talk about users 'exercising choice' and 'voting with their feet'), both of which are tied to what is probably an outdated model of power (i.e. who holds it and how can it be redistributed?).[58] A more contemporary approach to user involvement should be couched in terms of how power might be *generated* through co-production, which in the case of the MI centred on co-design, co-production of materials, co-leadership and mutual learning.

Co-production is a way of moving beyond the traditional rhetoric to bring service users more in partnership with providers and place them in a position of '*producing* public services as well as consuming or otherwise benefiting from them'.[59, 60] This approach to user involvement does not necessarily redress the power division between the 'provider' and 'user',[61] nor does it overcome the different motivations for involvement.

Co-design generally refers to involving service users in the planning and development of services. Bate and Robert coined the term 'experienced based co-design' to describe an innovate approach to service improvement using a range of methods to capture the experiences of both users and providers.[62] We consider this approach in Chapter 3 in relation to the MI.

Users' experiences and stories can be invaluable teaching material for staff, and can also assist others to make decisions about treatment choices. Through analysing a range of individual experiences

Ziebland and Herxheimer concluded that patient/user experiences should not be seen as a rival to the biomedical evidence base but rather as *part of* the overall evidence base which patients and carers should consider when making personal treatment choices.[63]

The involvement of users in education and training sees them switching from a more passive role to become more active in the eyes of the students/professionals. There is a tension in clinical education between ensuring that learners receive standardised training and assessment (e.g. the objective structured clinical evaluation with tightly scripted histories and symptoms) and offering 'real' patients in an unstandardised way.[64] Livingston and Cooper suggest that: 'involving patients as teachers has important educational benefits for learners: not only does it allow the acquisition of skills, but also it can change attitudes positively'[64] and Repper and Breeze comment: 'students report hearing real life experiences from consumer educators enhances their understanding'.[65] In Chapter 4 we consider examples of how stories of the user experience were used to educate both patients and staff in the MI.

Co-production of materials offers numerous potential opportunities for service users to have input to the design and dissemination of educational resources for staff and patients. Much emphasis has been placed on the quality and availability of such information. While it has been acknowledged that there is no shortage of information out there, 'the service user is left to dig it out for themselves and may not know what it is they need to know'.[66] The involvement of service users in the development of patient information tends to lead to resources that are more relevant, readable and understandable to patients than those developed by providers alone.[40] In Chapter 5 we consider how co-production played out in the MI.

As Chapter 6 describes in detail, co-opting service users into leadership positions can involve a range of activities from sitting on management or lay boards through to interview panels for new employees, but in order for these service users to participate effectively they must receive sufficient training to ensure that they are familiar with systems, processes and technical jargon or knowledge,[67] a requirement which may delay the decision-making process. Co-leadership and joint decision making raises the interesting issue of whether users might be involved to legitimise decisions that 'would have been made whether or not patients support them'[32] – a theme which we return to in Chapter 7.

Involving users in co-design and co-leadership entails the challenge of separating 'the user experience' from 'users' experiences'. In their research on user, involvement in the planning and delivery of adult mental health services in London, for example, Rutter et al. came across staff who criticised the 'inappropriate emotional outbursts' by users who 'tended to describe their own experiences of services during professional planning meetings'.[68] Participants may become frustrated because they are not able to discuss the issues which matter to them the most, perhaps because of the design of the interaction.[69] We describe how similar examples were addressed by the Modernisation Initiative (MI) teams in Chapter 6.

In summary, the literature on user involvement is philosophically and methodologically diverse, often critical, sometimes conflicting and replete with stories of unforeseen hurdles. Whilst we recommend that anyone setting out to involve users should familiarise themselves with key published research studies, these provide no easy formula for pulling off successful user involvement.

References

1. McIver A, Brocklehurst N. Public involvement: working for better health. *Nurs Stand* 1999;14(1):46–52.
2. Griffiths R. *The NHS Management Inquiry*. London: Department of Health and Social Security; 1983.
3. H.M. Government. *NHS and Community Care Act*. 1990.
4. NHS Management Executive. *Local voices. The Views of Local People in Purchasing for Health*. London: Department of Health; 1992.
5. Anonymous. *Final Report of the public inquiry into children's heart surgery at the Bristol Royal Infirmary 1984–1995*. Command Paper: CM 520. London: Stationery Office; 1998.
6. Smith J. *Safeguarding Patients—Lessons from the Past, Proposals for the Future (Shipman Inquiry)*. London: Stationery Office; 2004.
7. Redfern M. *Report of the Royal Liverpool Children's Inquiry*. London: Stationery Office; 1999.
8. Smith R. All changed, changed utterly. *BMJ* 1998; 316:1917–1918.
9. Bochel C, Bochel H, Somerville P, Worley C. Marginalised or enabled voices? 'User Participation' in policy and practice. *Soc Policy Soc* 2007; 7(2):201–210.
10. Department of Health. *In the Public Interest: Developing a Strategy for Public Participation in the NHS*. London: Stationery Office; 1998.
11. NHS Executive. *Patient and Public Involvement in the New NHS*. Leeds: Stationery Office; 1999.

12. Lorig K, Holman H. Arthritis self-management studies: a twelve-year review. *Health Educ Q* 1993; 20:17–28.
13. Lorig K. Partnerships between expert patients and physicians. *Lancet* 2002; 359:814–815.
14. Department of Health. *The Expert Patient: A New Approach to Chronic Disease Management for the Twenty-first Century*. London: Department of Health; 2001.
15. Donaldson L. Expert patients usher in a new era of opportunity for the NHS. *BMJ* 2003; 326:1279–1280.
16. Department of Health. *Saving Lives: Our Healthier Nation*. London: NHS Executive; 1999.
17. Clarke J. New Labour's citizens: activated, empowered, responsibilized, abandoned? *Crit Soc Policy* 2005; 25(4):447–463.
18. Greenhalgh T. Patient and public involvement in chronic illness: beyond the expert patient. *BMJ* 2009; 338:b49.
19. Fox NJ, Ward KJ, O'Rourke AJ. The 'expert patient': empowerment or medical dominance? The case of weight loss, pharmaceutical drugs and the Internet. *Soc Sci Med* 2005; 60(6):1299–1309.
20. Department of Health. *The NHS Plan*. London: NHS Executive; 2000.
21. Department of Health. *The NHS Plan: A Plan for Investment, A Plan for Reform*. London: NHS Executive; 2001.
22. Department of Health. *Shifting the Balance of Power Within the NHS*. London: The Stationery Office; 2001.
23. Baggott R. A funny thing happened on the way to the forum: reforming patient and public involvement in the NHS in England. *Public Adm* 2005; 83(3):533–551.
24. Department of Health. *Putting People First: A Shared Vision and Commitment to the Transformation of Adult Social Care*. London: The Stationery Office; 2007.
25. Department of Health. *Local Government and Public Involvement in Health Act*. London: The Stationery Office; 2007.
26. West D. Public LINks hit by delays in networking. *Health Serv J* 2008. Available at http://www.hsj.co.uk/public-links-hit-by-delays-in-networking/1894009.article.
27. Adamson D, Bromiley R. Community empowerment in practice. *Lessons from Communities First*. York: Joseph Rowntree Foundation; 2008.
28. Berwick DM. The science of improvement. *JAMA* 2008; 299(10):1182–1184.
29. Picker Institute. *Engaging Patients in Their Healthcare: How is the UK Doing Relative to Other Countries?* Oxford: Picker Institute Europe; 2006.
30. Florin D, Dixon J. Public involvement in health care. *BMJ* 2004; 328:159–161.

31. Bate P, Robert G. Toward more user-centric OD: lessons from the field of experience-based design and a case study. *J Appl Behav Sci* 2007; 43(1):41–66.
32. Crawford M, Rutter D, Manley C, Weaver T, Bhui K, Fulop N et al. Systematic review of involving patients in the planning and development of health care. *BMJ* 2002; 325:1263–1268.
33. Crawford M, Rutter D, Thelwall S. *User Involvement in Change Management: A Review of the Literature*. London: NHS Service Delivery and Organisation Programme; 2003.
34. Anonymous. *Involve and Together We Can. People and Participation*. London: Involve; 2006.
35. Foster J, Tyrell K, Cropper V, Junt N. Welcome to the team ... Service users in staff recruitment. *Drink and Drugs News* 2005; 21 March www.drinkanddrugs.net.
36. Simpson E, House A, Barkham M. *A Guide to Involving Users and Carers in Mental Health Service Planning, Delivery or Research: A Health Technology Approach*. Leeds: Academic Unit of Psychiatry and Behavioral Sciences, University of Leeds; 2002.
37. Beresford P. User involvement in research: exploring the challenges. *Nursing Times Research* 2003; 8(1):36–46.
38. Boote J, Telford R, Cooper C. Consumer involvement in health research: a review and research agenda. *Health Policy* 2002; 61:213–236.
39. NHS Confederation. *Future Leadership; Reforming Leadership Development ... Again*. London: NHS Confederation Publications; 2009.
40. Nilsen ES, Myrhaug HT, Johansen M, Oliver S, Oxman AD. Methods of consumer involvement in developing healthcare policy and research, clinical practice guidelines and patient information material. *Cochrane Database Syst Rev* 2006; 3:CD004563.
41. Beresford P. 'Service user': regressive or liberatory terminology? *Disabil Soc* 2005; 20(4):469–477.
42. Peck E, Barker I. Users as partners in mental health – ten years of experience. *J Interprof Care* 1997; 11:269–277.
43. Crossley ML, Crossley N. 'Patient' voices, social movements and the habitus; how psychiatric survivors 'speak out'. *Soc Sci Med* 2001; 52(10):1477–1489.
44. Stickley T. Should service user involvement be consigned to history? A critical realist perspective. *J Psychiatr Ment Health Nurs* 2006; 13: 570–577.
45. Greener I. Choice and voice – a review. *Soc Policy Soc* 2007; 7(2): 255–265.
46. Main T. The hospital as a therapeutic institution. *Bull Menninger Clin* 1946; 10:66–70.
47. Arnstein S. A ladder of citizen participation. *J Am Inst Plann* 1969; 35:216–224.

48. Tritter JQ, McCallum A. The snakes and ladders of user involvement: moving beyond Arnstein. *Health Policy* 2006; 76(2):156–168.
49. Illich I. *Disabling Professions*. London: Marion Boyars; 1977.
50. Department of Health Care Services Improvement Partnership. *Reward and Recognition: The Principles and Practice of Service User Payment and Reimbursement in Health and Social Care*. London: Stationery Office; 2006.
51. Carr S. Participation, power, conflict and change: Theorizing dynamics of service user participation in the social care system of England and Wales. *Crit Soc Policy* 2007; 27(2):266–276.
52. Edelman M. *Politics as Symbolic Action*. New York: Free Press; 1971.
53. Republic of South Africa. *A Guide to Revitalise Batho Pele*. Johannesburg: Department of Public Service and Administration; 2007.
54. Greenhalgh T, Wessely S. 'Health for me': a sociocultural analysis of healthism in the middle classes. *Br Med Bull* 2004; 69:197–213.
55. Greenhalgh T, Heath I. *Measuring Quality in the Therapeutic Relationship*. London: Kings Fund; 2010.
56. McLean A. Empowerment and the psychiatric consumer/ex-patient movement in the United States: contradictions, crisis and change. *Soc Sci Med* 1995; 40(8):1053–1081.
57. Carr S, Robbins D. *The Implementation of Individual Budget Schemes in Adult Social Care*. London: Social Care Institute for Excellence Research (Briefing no. 20); 2009.
58. Hardy C, Clegg SR. Some dare call it power. In: Clegg SR, Hardy C, Nord WR, editors. *Handbook of Organizational Studies*. London: Sage; 1996; 622–641.
59. Alford J. A public management road less travelled: clients as co-producers of public services. *Aust J Public Adm* 1998; 57(4):128–137.
60. Needham C. Realising the potential of co-production: negotiating improvements in public services. *Soc Policy Soc* 2008; 7(2):221–231.
61. Barnes D, Carpenter J, Bailey D. Partnerships with service users in interprofessional education for community mental health: a case study. *J Interprof Care* 2000; 14(2):189–200.
62. Bate SP, Robert G. *Bringing User Experience to Healthcare Improvement*. Oxford: Radcliffe; 2007.
63. Ziebland S, Herxheimer A. How patients' experiences contribute to decision making: illustrations from DIPEx (personal experiences of health and illness). *J Nurs Manag* 2008; 16(4):433–439.
64. Livingston G, Cooper C. User and carer involvement in mental health training. *Adv Psychiatr Treat* 2004; 10:84–92.
65. Repper J, Breeze J. User and carer involvement in the training and education of health professionals: a review of the literature. *Int J Nurs Stud* 2007; 44(3):511–519.

66. Swain D, Ellins J, Coulter A, Heron P, Howell E, McGee H et al. *Accessing Information About Health and Social Care Services*. Oxford: Picker Institute; 2007.

67. Fudge N, Wolfe CD, McKevitt C. Assessing the promise of user involvement in health service development: ethnographic study. *BMJ* 2008; 336(7639):313–317.

68. Rutter D, Manley C, Weaver T, Crawford MJ, Fulop N. Patients or partners? Case studies of user involvement in the planning and delivery of adult mental health services in London. *Soc Sci Med* 2004; 58(10):1973–1984.

69. Hodge S. Participation, discourse and power: a case study in service user involvement. *Crit Soc Policy* 2005; 25:164–179.

CHAPTER 3

Experience-based co-design

Vikki Pearce[1], Paula Baraitser[2], Gaynor Smith[3]
& Trisha Greenhalgh[4]
[1]NHS Tower Hamlets, London, UK
[2]King's College Hospital, NHS Foundation Trust, London, UK
[3]End of Life Care Programme, Modernisation Initiative, St. Thomas'
Hospital, London, UK
[4]Queen Mary, University of London, London, UK

The term 'experience-based co-design' was coined by Paul Bate and Glenn Robert to describe an innovative approach to service improvement. The principle is to employ a range of methods creatively and adaptively to capture the experiences of both patients and staff, and use this special form of expertise (the experience of those involved in the process) to redesign all or part of that process to make it more fit for purpose. As Bate and Robert emphasise in their book, experience-based co-design deliberately draws out the subjective, personal feelings that patients, carers and staff experience at crucial points in the care pathway and enables all stakeholders to then work together to bring about sustained improvements in those experiences.[1] This approach has been used both in healthcare (see examples of experience-based co-design in improving services for cancer,[2] chronically sick adolescents,[3] and people with dementia and their carers[4]) and more widely (see, for example, the use of experience-based co-design in the development of social housing[5]).

The modernisation initiative (MI) included a number of subprojects in which experience-based co-design was a central feature of efforts to involve users. In this chapter, we describe four contrasting examples of this approach: mystery shoppers in sexual health, whole-systems events in kidney services, focus groups of 'seldom

User Involvement in Health Care, 1st edition. Edited by Trisha Greenhalgh,
Charlotte Humphrey and Fran Woodard. © 2011 Blackwell Publishing Ltd.

heard' service users in sexual health and care pathway redesign in stroke services. We then draw on these very different examples to offer some principles for applying experience-based co-design – especially the challenge of engaging and retaining an appropriate cohort of users.

Example 1: Mystery shoppers

One approach to user involvement that generated much interest outside the MI was the sexual health MI's use of 'mystery shoppers' – patients or ex-patients who were trained to visit the service incognito and write up their experiences of different parts of the system.[6,7] All the service providers knew about the mystery shopper project in principle, but of course did not know the users or how they would present themselves.

The mystery shopper project was partly inspired by a successful local project in which women 'training associates' were recruited to teach medical students pelvic examinations while playing the role of patients. Although this initiative predated the MI, it inspired a key MI work stream in which participants from a broad range of social and ethnic groups and sexual orientations were recruited and trained to visit services and provide detailed feedback on pre-specified quality indicators.

The mystery shoppers were paid to present with one of several standardised stories to different parts of the sexual health services. They received training on the standards that they should be able to expect from the services and were encouraged to provide constructive criticism. After each round of visits they met with a known member of the sexual health MI team to provide feedback on their experience and discuss possible solutions to any problems identified. This method enabled the collection of quantitative and qualitative data on actual experience of service provision and provided consistent, regular feedback both to identify problems and monitor the impact of improvements over time.

Feedback from mystery shoppers was seen as providing important and credible insights into the experience of using services and was generally well received by clinic staff. Such feedback was used extensively in the design of the new sexual health service. It was mystery shopper data that led to close attention being paid to reducing waiting times and number of visits, building a culture in which service users' privacy and dignity are respected by all staff and improving the physical surroundings of the clinic so that the waiting was more tolerable. The mystery shoppers remained engaged because they were well supported and could see that they were making a difference to the services they visited.

Nevertheless there were considerable challenges associated with this approach, including the resources required to train, supervise and support the cohort of mystery shoppers and ensure that they included representatives from different client groups; the risk that as mystery shoppers themselves became 'experts' on the service, their assessments would become more critical, thereby potentially masking improvements over time; the complex nature of data generated by mystery shopper visits; and the concern of a minority of staff that the approach was in an ethical 'grey zone'.

The sexual health MI produced a guide to involving users as mystery shoppers: '*Mystery Shopping in Sexual Health: A toolkit for delivery*', available as a free download from http://www.gsttcharity.org.uk/pdfs/mystery.pdf.[8]

Example 2: Whole systems events to improve kidney services

Events where patients and staff meet together to map out all the steps in the care pathway are potentially powerful change tools. Mapping the pathway from the user's perspective can provide staff with insights into how patients and carers experience the service. Such events may also enable staff who work on separate parts of the pathway to see the pathway in its entirety.

The 'whole-systems event' was a structured one-day meeting between service users and staff. The kidney MI held 13 such events throughout the 3-year MI period, each one bringing groups of patients together with all of those involved in their care, including ward cleaners, porters, managers and clinical staff. Over time, a structure developed that all participants felt worked well. In the morning, patients and professionals worked in separate groups to share experience of what worked and what could be improved. Then everyone had lunch together. After lunch, the groups came together to compare perspectives, discuss problems and generate possible improvements. The last part of the day was spent in mixed groups of patients, carers and professionals, each working on a specific issue to develop an action plan. At this point people were invited to become involved in ongoing service improvement work.

After the event, everyone who had attended received a letter summarising the discussion and action points.

Whole-systems events had the advantage of bringing staff and service users together in a format where everyone knew that the goal was to change the way the service was organised and delivered. Participants were usually committed and keen before they arrived, and the events were typically characterised by a sense of creative energy and a clear focus on the patient experience. Events were seen as helping staff to understand patients' and carers' concerns in a way that is quite different from one-to-one consultations: they get to 'know what they don't know'. The fact that staff were giving up their personal time to be there sent a very powerful message to patients and carers that their views were being taken seriously.

A lot can be achieved in a day, especially if those who attend are broadly representative of the wider patient population and their experience is fully and faithfully captured and fed into the redesign process. These, of course, are big 'ifs'. In the kidney MI, most of the whole systems events were well attended by a broad group of service users and produced important insights for redesigning the service. But across the MI more widely, other sub-projects had varying success with organising whole systems events. In some cases, the users recruited either did not turn up or did not seem to represent the views of all those who used the service. Once or twice, staff were concerned that what they were 'capturing' was little more than the personal agenda of single-issue campaigners. At other times, the concerns of patients seemed to be beyond the remit of the team that had come together to address the pathway – an issue which we take up later in this chapter.

The kidney MI produced a guide to running such events, *'Improving Services by Involving Patients, Carers and Staff'*, available as a free download from http://www.gsttcharity.org.uk/pdfs/kidney_whole_system_event_toolkit.pdf.[9]

Example 3: Redesigning the physical environment of a sexual health clinic

In this example, we describe efforts of the sexual health MI team to modernise the clinic environment so as to make the service more accessible and acceptable. Early interviews with both users and staff had identified the physical characteristics of the clinics as contributing to a poor user experience. The different clinics across the two boroughs varied in quality. At best, they took the form of a conventional hospital outpatient department. At worst, they were poorly designed, dark, old-fashioned and in disrepair. This compounded the feelings of shame and anxiety that many users experienced. It was clear that redesign of the *service* should include redesign of the *clinic environment* – and that more than a lick of paint would be needed.

The challenge in sexual health was that 'users' of the service tend to have only a brief encounter with it – and they may not wish to be recognised or approached as a 'sexual health service user'. This made recruiting anyone – let alone a representative sample – extremely difficult, but staff were encouraged to come up with creative solutions and pursue them. It was suggested that waiting rooms might be an obvious place to make contact with users. However, waiting rooms are often uncomfortable places associated with the stress of long waits, apprehension about the consultation and a lack of confidentiality. Even approaching individual users in this setting to invite them to move to a more private place for a conversation about potential involvement can be problematic.

Staff addressed this challenge by producing two large paintings – one of a tree and one of a brick wall – which were attached to the waiting room wall. One facilitator led a discussion about the clinic environment while the other approached people waiting for their appointment and invited them to write positive comments on leaf shaped 'post-it' notes, which were stuck to the branches of the tree, and negative comments on brick shaped 'post-it' notes, which they attached to the brick wall. Encouraging people to leave their seats to attach the notes and to participate in the discussion seemed to generate a positive atmosphere in a previously silent waiting room. During the session, everyone was invited to a larger event where similar techniques would be used to discuss other aspects of the service.

The main point of this activity was the opportunity to experience what engagement might be like, not the data that were collected. To an audience of sexual health service users who were *potentially* interested in user involvement it demonstrated that people did not have to talk about their specific health needs in order to contribute to the co-design process.

In the definitive co-design events, staff used a series of pictures of innovative and exciting architecture (not all from healthcare) to stimulate thinking among service users on the design of a new clinic. Some users thought that these idealised designs were 'too nice' and would encourage people to use the services excessively. Others worried that the 'nice' environments would be ruined by children or other attenders (a café would be welcome but spilled drinks would spoil the waiting room). There was a huge diversity of views on whether each specific design was attractive or not, and discussions on these were often lively (and sometimes chaotic).

After several such sessions, some key design principles were identified on which most people agreed. Examples of these were:

- Making the first step into the building easy by having a welcoming entrance;
- Revealing the interior in stages, so that passers-by might see into the building but could not see people waiting inside;
- 'Visible but invisible' – i.e. striking a balance between (on the one hand) making the service prominent and easy to identify so that people can find it, and (on the other hand) having an entrance that is discrete so people do not feel too embarrassed to get through the door; and
- Having a light airy environment with strong bright colours and a modern feel.

These 'concepts' were given to the architects, who generated a range of possible design solutions. A number of subsequent events were held with staff, users in the waiting room and experienced mystery shoppers (see Example 1 above) to discuss the potential designs. At each stage the options were narrowed down and the questions asked became more focused. This funnelling process enabled everyone to contribute before agreeing the final design. After the new clinic was opened, mystery shoppers were asked to provide feedback, which confirmed that the new environment was well received by users representing a range of age, gender, ethnicity and sexual orientation. (Figure 3.1)

The above examples raise a number of issues and challenges which are common to all or most efforts to involve users in co-design. We discuss these below.

Challenge 1: Attracting a representative cohort of users

Given that there are so many patients in the system, it might come as a surprise that engaging a cohort of users to help with a co-design

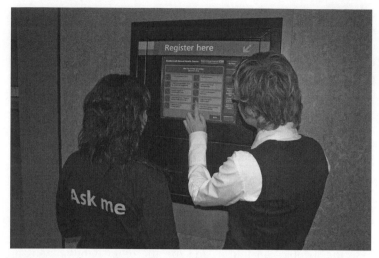

Figure 3.1 Redesigned sexual health clinic with touch screen registration.

or redesign initiative can be difficult. But being a *patient* in the clinic or on the ward is a completely different role from being a participant in co-design, and the latter must be systematically recruited. 'Getting hold of users' can be divided into four steps: identification, engagement, recruitment and retention.

In the *identification* phase, you need to define a group of users or potential users of the service. One way of refining your target group might be to set out what you want users to contribute. Depending on the group identified, the method of *engagement* will vary. People who are already known to service providers and actively use services, such as those with a diagnosis of high blood pressure or established kidney disease, are relatively easy to identify and recruit. Others, including *potential* users who have never been in contact or past users who are no longer in contact with services, are more difficult to find.

The project team found it invaluable to have a register of service users who could be called up and asked if they were free for a forthcoming initiative. Sometimes we selected users for specific tasks or projects because they either had skills in this area, or we knew it was something they felt strongly about. At other times, we invited all the users on the list and allowed them to self-select.

The *engagement* phase is not simply the initial approach to recruit users at the outset of the project. It is not always sufficient to engage a fixed group of people at the start of the initiative and work with these for the duration of the project. In most of the MI sub-projects, we planned for new people to be engaged periodically throughout the work. Some users will opt not to be involved, become too unwell to continue involvement or move onto a different stage of treatment and cease their involvement with the service undergoing improvement. Also, consulting the same people over and over again may lead to overfamiliarisation with the service and the development of 'expert user' status. On the positive side, this generates a group who have detailed knowledge of the service improvement process and the confidence to engage with it, but on the negative side there will inevitably be a loss of the 'fresh' perspective and new ideas. Furthermore, a small group of service users may not have knowledge of all aspects of a service, and 'new blood' tends to increase the range of contributions.

Almost all the sub-projects in the MI reported a common finding – that *recruitment* of users was far more time-consuming and labour-intensive than they had initially anticipated, as this quote shows:

> So we set three dates, each about a month apart. And the 200 people that said they would come and contribute further to the work, I think they were written to in the first instance and then they were telephoned. And they were followed up with telephone calls, three times I think before they were crossed off the list. From the 200 we wrote to them, we rang them, we rang them, we rang them, we offered to pay them and 91 of them actually came to an event. (Programme Manager, sexual health MI).

This general finding was particularly true when staff made special efforts to overcome recruitment bias – the well-described problem of gaining unrepresentative samples when 'convenience' methods are used. Sending an email to a user discussion group or asking selected 'approachable' patients in clinic is likely to bias the sample in favour of the articulate, information-rich and compliant end of the user spectrum.

But overcoming recruitment bias can be an uphill struggle. The sexual health MI, for example, sought to gather information from large numbers of users about their current experience of services. The aim was to understand the variation in experience among a user group that was known to be diverse. Over a 1-month period they recruited participants by running 'ad hoc' focus groups in clinic waiting rooms. This gave people a taste of the involvement process and meant that the invitation to take part reached hundreds of people. This approach recruited a wide range of current users but did not reach past users or those who chose *not* to visit this clinic.

In some cases an *intentionally* 'biased' sample (i.e. purposively oversampling from groups with particular needs) may be justified. For example, within sexual health services sex workers may have particular clinical and/or social needs but these may remain hidden unless a specific effort is made to recruit this group. Similarly, limited English speakers may be excluded from most consultation events unless they are identified and catered for.

Recruitment bias may sometimes be overcome not through systematic 'statistical sampling' from the outset but by creatively extending from what is known to be a biased initial sample. For example, the sexual health MI wished to work with mystery shoppers who would be prepared to undergo a clinical examination as part of their mystery shopper consultation. Initially we were concerned that our pool of service users would not be prepared to do this so we recruited from an existing group of women who were trained to teach pelvic examination to medical students from the patient perspective. This group were very comfortable about going through an internal examination for training or evaluation purposes but they were older than the average service users and unusually comfortable in clinical environments. As the mystery shopper programme became more established, we offered this role to a range of service users, including many young people. We learnt, somewhat to our surprise, that a wide range of people were happy to take on this role once its purpose had been explained. Two sisters became pivotal in this programme. They had been involved in the MI from an early stage and became and remained a key channel through which the MI communicated with a large number of others. They supported the recruitment of other mystery shoppers through their friendship groups and although the MI had the telephone numbers of that wider group, other users did not tend to respond unless contacted directly by one of the sisters.

In some services, especially those for long-term conditions, health professionals may be willing to ask patients attending clinic to user involvement activities. Some users are well known to their clinicians, and we found that kidney patients in particular often see the same clinician regularly for many years. Recruitment by clinicians creates an opportunity for a conversation about involvement to happen but decisions about who to invite will be influenced by the clinician's perception of the patient's ability to contribute. Similarly the patient's willingness to participate might be influenced by their dependent status.

Some clinicians may (consciously or unconsciously) approach users who are likely to support the status quo, and those users may also be more likely to accept the invitation. On the other hand, clinicians who seek to drive change may 'hand pick' patients who have an axe to grind! One consultant involved in the programme reflected on how long he had known his patients and the opportunities this presented to approach them about becoming involved:

'... the only way to get away from me would be either dying or I retire. And some of the patients, they've known me since 1979'. He also reflected on why he invited a particular patient to participate: *'Yes. I've known H quite a while, and H was known as a difficult patient. Actually I had a great deal of time for the way that H had actually controlled his treatment to fit in with what he wanted to do'.*

Another possible way to recruit users who are no longer in regular contact with the service is to use a register and send a mailshot. However, under the Data Protection Act (see http://www.ico.gov.uk/), approaching people in this way may only be done if patients have given explicit permission to be contacted. In the stroke MI, a well-maintained register of all people who had had a stroke in the area was available, and everyone on the register who had given prior consent was invited to be involved. An important problem with this approach is that if the registers are of 'past' patients rather than those actively in contact with the service, there is a possibility that some people approached will have died. *'That's happened a few times. And that's been very painful for all concerned obviously'* (Service improvement facilitator, stroke MI).

One important route for recruitment is through community and voluntary organisations which could provide access to groups of service users not easily identified through healthcare provision. There is a wide range of these organisations from small local groups to national organisations and each has its own culture and focus, which set the parameters of engagement. The stroke MI team relied heavily on voluntary groups to recruit people who had experienced strokes and who were interested in user involvement. They contacted a huge range of voluntary organisations, many of who were not specifically targeting those with strokes, and recruited 60–70 volunteers in this way. Similarly, the sexual health MI gathered feedback from commercial sex workers via a local support group to check that the service redesign plans (see Example 3 above) would meet their needs. It is crucial to think creatively about how to access users beyond those most likely to volunteer or the 'majority' users of the service.

When recruiting and retaining users, it is important to take account of how their illness or disability may affect their ability to participate and design the involvement approach accordingly. Some service users are more likely to have time, opportunity and motivation to be involved because of the nature of their condition. Kidney patients on dialysis spend hours in the unit every week and some though, not all of them, may be able to use this time in some way to help improve their experience. They may also be keen to do so, because they expect to benefit personally over a number of years. But kidney failure is an exhausting and demanding condition, and chronic fatigue may limit even the most well-motivated patient's ability to contribute on a regular basis. Conversely, many users of sexual health services will visit clinics only briefly and intermittently and may be reluctant to identify with them. For people living with stroke, physical or communication difficulties associated with the condition may act as barriers to engaging in service co-design. However sexual health service users are much less likely to have chronic ill health and once recruited may be able to participate actively and enthusiastically.

The decision to engage or not may coincide with personal issues such as work/childcare commitments and the opportunities for social engagement that involvement affords. These factors should influence the choice of engagement opportunities. Those with extensive work commitments may prefer on-line discussion groups, those with limited social opportunities may value interactive events and those with childcare responsibilities will value free childcare at user consultation events and meetings.

An alternative approach, which we employed in some settings, is to work directly with individuals whose task is to represent the concerns of wider groups. For example, voluntary organisation representatives were invited to meetings to plan service developments for sexual health services. They were highly articulate and very vocal as advocates for the needs of specific groups of users. This sometimes became difficult, if they saw their role as campaigning for particular priority groups rather than all the users of the service.

Challenge 2: Making involvement achievable and worthwhile for users

During the course of the MI we learnt that some users have more time, energy and commitment than others, and that it was important to be flexible so that users could choose what they felt willing and able to do at any particular time. Clarity about what was expected in terms of time and type of input was essential for gaining commitment. Whether users chose to be involved generally depended on their availability, their interest in the topic, the skills they felt they had to contribute, the time commitment and a 'what's in it for me?' factor. If being involved was perceived to be easy, enjoyable and fulfilling, and especially if users gained personally in some way, recruiting and retaining them was much easier, as the quote below shows.

> . . .*people involved in the stroke programme variously told us that they appreciated meeting other people with similar experiences to them – a particular example was younger people who had had a stroke and were parenting – valued the opportunity to learn more about their condition in the course of the involvement, others found it something enjoyable to do with their time to get out and have some company, others putting something back, making a difference for other people who came along after them.* (Service improvement lead, stroke MI)

Box 3.1 shows some benefits of user involvement from the user's perspective.

Our experience suggests that whatever the specific project, attempts to get users involved are more likely to succeed if people see that there is some point in participating (i.e. that *they personally* have something to contribute that will actually make a difference to something that matters to them) and if the experience of involvement will be interesting, enjoyable, rewarding and not too onerous. The MI teams learnt that targeting invitations carefully can help enormously. In the early days of the kidney MI, for example, letters were sent out to 3000 kidney patients inviting them to attend a whole-systems event with the rather vague aim of 'identifying ways to improve services for people with kidney disease'. Of the 3000, only 25 people (fewer than 1%) attended the event. But on the second occasion, the team adopted a much more focused approach. They invited only 200 people, all of whom were on the kidney transplant waiting list, and the letters said that the

Box 3.1 Possible benefits of user involvement to users

- Social interaction, meeting other people with similar problems
- Gaining knowledge about their condition
- Learning about the available health services and how to access them
- Learning how to manage their condition
- Learning broader skills, e.g. presentation skills, basic research techniques, participating in meetings
- Payment and/or benefits in kind (e.g. high quality refreshments)
- Fulfilment (a feeling that they are 'making a difference')
- Giving positive feedback to a valued service

event would be concerned specifically with improving communication about transplant issues. Out of 200 people contacted, 60 (30%) came to the event.

In this socio-economically deprived area, payment appeared to be an important incentive for participation. Sexual health service users were routinely paid around £10 per hour (2007 prices) for their participation in consultation and redesign initiatives – a level which generally did not interfere with their state benefits. The programme staff felt this was an important aspect of valuing the contribution users were making to the redesign process, and preferred cash to vouchers as they felt that users should be allowed to choose how and where to spend their money. Occasionally, the 'carrot' of a cash payment led to users from relatively hard-to-reach minorities turning up with several friends, leading some staff to feel that some users were 'taking advantage' of the user involvement process.

Kidney and stroke service users were not routinely paid for their involvement, and some felt that they would not want to be paid because they were 'putting something back' or contributing to a service from which they intended to benefit. This highlights, perhaps, some interesting socio-demographic differences between the users in the different MI projects, and also shows how the long-term nature of stroke and kidney problems means that relationships between users and staff are built on different foundations. Whether and how people get paid for making a contribution is one of the inherent tensions of user involvement which is discussed further in Chapter 7.

Challenge 3: Preparing users

We found that we needed to pay close attention to providing information about the user involvement process and ensuring that all parties understood what was expected of them, as this quote shows:

> *Despite our best efforts, some patients came along not having a clue what they were coming to. So, from that point of view it might have either been daunting or a waste of their time . . . . . . I think you have to word things very carefully.* (Service improvement lead)

Some of this preparation work can be done at the events themselves. In the whole systems events (see Example 2 above), the entire morning of a one-day event was given over to preparing users and staff for the afternoon session of working together on a plan for service redesign. This morning session included discussion about *how* to work together and making this a safe process for both users and staff. Users were given an introduction to National Health Service (NHS) structures and terminology to enable them to articulate their concerns, and staff were supported not to be defensive about the feedback they might receive from users. Users practised giving feedback in a constructive way.

Sometimes, 'preparing' users may potentially affect their input to the improvement process. In the initial stages of the mystery shopper programme, for example, we were anxious about how the visits might go and invested in extensive preparation for the mystery shoppers. We felt we were always balancing the tension of giving them enough information to prepare them properly and leaving them to their own devices so as to give a more authentic 'user experience'. We gradually became more confident in distinguishing what information to give them in advance and what we expected them to find out themselves. So for example, initially we gave out leaflets and detailed information about the services, but as time went on we expected them to find this information (or not) for themselves – and if they did not find it, we were alerted to the need to make it more visible.

Another aspect of preparation is clarity about the need to be punctual and reliable in attending meetings and events and about the level and type of input needed. Some service users do not have strictly timetabled lives (or even diaries or watches), and may not be skilled at articulating their views either verbally or in writing. However, we quickly found that user involvement was extremely difficult to achieve if no expectations were placed on users to turn up at agreed times for agreed inputs.

For example, over time we developed a set of terms and conditions for the mystery shoppers. Initially we invited people to come to a briefing meeting, and at this meeting we would allocate them a number of visits each. We learnt through experience that not all mystery shoppers would complete their visits and not all shoppers who completed their visits would complete their reports and submit them on time. This resulted in some services getting reports for a very small number of visits – which had limited value to the providers of those services. Also some of the mystery shoppers submitted very brief reports that conveyed little of the user experience. The terms and conditions we developed (expressed as an informal 'contract' between the service and the mystery shopper) specified what we expected from people taking part in the programme (visits must be completed and reports submitted on time) and also what they could expect from us (support during visits, prompt payment, references, further visits). Very occasionally, we did not invite people back because they failed to meet these conditions. In the sexual health project we also developed similar informal contracts at the start of consultation events or focus groups so as to make the rules of engagement explicit.

Preparation includes helping users and staff develop realistic expectations of what can and cannot be achieved via a particular exercise. Not all suggestions for improvement will be feasible and implementing many of them may take a long time. For example, the kidney MI found that the poor reliability of the hospital transport was seen as a priority for service improvement by many hospital patients, but dealing with this problem was beyond the remit of the staff attending the event. The most they could do was pass on the users' concerns and ideas to the transport team – and some patients remained dissatisfied at the lack of progress in this area (perhaps reasonably since the initiative had been billed as a 'whole systems' event).

Challenge 4: Preparing and including staff

Some of our attempts to involve users undoubtedly faltered because staff were poorly prepared and failed to understand either their own role in the user involvement exercise or the users' role. We found that staff who were engaged and positive about the idea of user involvement before the consultation began tended to work with users to find creative solutions to challenges such as health and safety regulations and clinical governance issues. But those who either did not understand or did not value the idea of user involvement sometimes used these service constraints to block user led development.

For example, a consultation with users about the waiting room environment generated a number of practical suggestions about refreshment facilities and improvements to the furnishings and decorations. Failure to engage all staff in this process resulted in them being unsupportive of the proposed changes. When asked to comment on the users' suggestions, one staff member said:

> *I have tried [providing] magazines – they steal and vandalise them. Many clients bring their own food and drink to the clinic and leave the remnants all over the floor and the chairs for someone else to clear up. It can be quite disgusting at times. So, as for drink and food and a nice, blue carpet? I don't think so!* (Receptionist)

Although clinic staff were consulted on the plans, they were not involved (and their views were not prioritised) to anything like the same extent as users. So, for example, the new design did not include a staff room. The modernisation of the service required staff to take on new roles and work in different ways, and some of them would have been a lot more enthusiastic if consideration had also been given to more direct staff benefits. We learnt from this that it is best to invest in engaging staff before users are approached, if only to reassure staff that their views are also valued and would be fed into the redesign process.

Challenge 5: Identifying problems

Even though users are 'experts' in the experience of a service, the process of redesign or co-design can be hard to operationalise. In particular, we found that 'identifying problems' was surprisingly difficult. Service users may be reluctant – perhaps at an unconscious level – to identify deficiencies in services on which they are dependent. They may have limited knowledge of what is considered 'best practice', and they may be accustomed to receiving care that does not meet prevailing standards. Finally, they may be unaware of what alternatives are available.

For example, when sexual health service users were first asked for feedback on the clinical consultation, they volunteered information about the friendliness of the clinical staff and their general approach but made no comment on issues such as privacy. When they were informed about clinical standards on providing clients with privacy to undress they started to comment on this and revealed that they would indeed value greater privacy. When asked about the waiting room environment, many felt it would be inappropriate to have anything other than rows of chairs in neutral colours and an essentially unwelcoming atmosphere, otherwise people might overuse the service or vandalise furniture. But when they became aware that a major problem in sexual health was failure of vulnerable groups to access services, they were strongly supportive of a more welcoming and comfortable waiting area.

We found that even when users were clear in their own minds about what needed to be improved, skilled facilitation was essential to get them to articulate their views. People typically needed both permission and encouragement to constructively criticise. In addition, some way had to be found to convey expected standards of best practice without prejudicing users' assessments of what was important to *them*. For example, we developed an introductory session for the sexual health mystery shoppers which encouraged constructive input, and also raised awareness of available standards in terms of staff attitudes, waiting times, waiting environments and information provision about services and health problems.

There are a number of established approaches to 'kick starting' a co-design process. Analysing complaints is one obvious place to start. Most services collect complaints anyway and a response to these is mandatory within the NHS. But only certain groups of users have the confidence and skills to use the complaints procedure. Moreover, we found that staff were often dismissive of problems identified via complaints, arguing that they did not represent the majority of users' views. Other methods for problem identification include suggestions boxes or patient satisfaction questionnaires, all of which may be useful for kick-starting a redesign event.

The question of how and when to survey service users is highly controversial. Surveys allow for rapid consultation of large numbers of patients and carers, but whilst samples can be large they are not necessarily representative. They also have well-documented limitations as tools for capturing people's experience of service use – chiefly that people who return completed questionnaires differ systematically from those who do not.[10] In addition, administering questionnaires and gaining complete and accurate data is a sophisticated task which if not done to a high standard will result in poor quality data from which few conclusions can be drawn.

For example, the sexual health MI within the MI attempted to access a wide range of potential users by paying voluntary organisations representing groups with particular service needs, e.g. mental health service users, gay men, to administer questionnaires to their members. Although this drew a reasonable response rate, we found a high proportion of missing data and it was often difficult to tell how the data had been collected. We learnt that whilst partnering with user organisations to help identify problems is a good idea in principle, there needs to be clear agreement in terms of the quality of data expected.

We did, however, encounter many examples of small-scale user surveys which staff perceived as easy to administer and analyse and which contributed directly to immediate and cost-neutral improvements to the service, as the following quote illustrates:

the waiting area at the unit – all the chairs were positioned kind of facing the toilet door, which ... you know, just not very nice being watched when you were going in and out and that sort of thing, which I don't know if any of the staff had actually thought of. (Kidney dialysis unit, service user)

Surveys were not the only form of quantitative data which were useful in the problem identification phase of redesign. Often, both users and staff were aware of a problem which had not been systematically documented or measured. This was the case with dialysis waiting times in the kidney programme, as this quote shows:

I think [there was] a general impression and understanding that things weren't running quite smoothly up there and yes an awareness that there were extended waits and it's a very busy unit and the flow of patients wasn't being managed as well as it could be. But, you know, at that point there wasn't the data to sort of back it up. So the first point was data collection. And when I did that it just involved sort of shadowing patients, arriving and going in for dialysis and coming out again. (Service improvement facilitator)

The data collection on waiting times confirmed subjective impressions and shocked both patients and staff. The quantitative data seemed to spur a change to the service in a more or less direct way:

Once we'd got the data, the solution was kind of obvious in terms of going from a first come first served system to a scheduled slot. (Service improvement facilitator)

Challenge 6: Generating potential solutions

We found that the best methods for generating solutions were often different from those needed to identify problems. The key task in the former is stimulating creative thinking and moving both users and staff beyond their past experience and (often) expectations for how the service might be run.

Finding aspects of the service that are already working well, and bringing insights from these to bear on problems in other parts of the service (as in 'what can we learn from the positive experience in clinic A which might solve a problem identified in clinic B?') is one way to help generate solutions. We found that users involved in the sexual health mystery shopping project soon built up a broad knowledge base about the range of provision across local services, and were able to encourage sharing of good practice.

Whilst surveys can be useful for identifying problems (see previous section), they are less useful for generating ideas or offering solutions. The kidney MI user survey of dialysis services identified that some patients found the unit environment too warm and some found it too cold. This was useful information on the problem, but further work was required to think about how these different temperature preferences could be accommodated within a single unit.

If radical solutions are needed, people often need encouragement to abandon their preconceptions of how a service 'ought' to run. We took some service users to visit examples of attractive health service architecture or innovative clinical practice, so as to help them move beyond a perception that the current local model was the only one available. In another example, the kidney MI used a series of visits with users and clinicians to a nocturnal dialysis programme in Holland to stimulate user demand for this service and answer questions and concerns from clinicians and patients. This was a powerful approach as it seemed to consolidate a shared vision of how this service could be offered. One of the staff who went on the second visit commented:

> *Well I think just in terms of the sort of discussion we had, it was multifaceted, people had different approaches, different agendas and were asking different questions, so we covered a lot of ground. Probably more importantly it was kind of gelling in terms of the shared experience and then going on from there, we were all on the same page, it wasn't that some people had this experience and got this extra information and others were still in the dark.* (Service improvement lead)

Interestingly, we found that users tended to be conservative in the solutions they proposed themselves but often greeted innovative ideas from elsewhere with great enthusiasm.

Another approach to stimulating creative thinking was using examples from outside health care. For example in preparation for a discussion on the refurbishment of a new sexual health service, users were taken to visit a community centre, an architect's practice and looked at the design of a high-profile sports store on Regent Street. All these buildings illustrated imaginative approaches to the challenge of creating a public space that was highly accessible from the street but also clearly separated from it. Whilst these designs did not influence the design of the sexual health centre directly, we believe they enabled users and staff to think imaginatively about the entrance and street frontage to the successfully redesigned sexual health centre.

Challenge 7: Selecting solutions and deciding next steps

In some circumstances, solutions offered by service users and staff in co-design initiatives were unworkable, unaffordable or impossible based on legitimate external considerations such as local or national policy, availability of premises, level of investment required and the need to ensure (and be seen to provide) equity in service provision. Often, much work had to be done to align blue-skies thinking with the constraints of what was practically possible.

There was also the problem of micropolitics. We found that even when users had come up with clear suggestions for change, their suggestions were sometimes rejected by staff for 'technical' reasons (such as health and safety) or because particular staff perceived that the new service model would impact negatively on their own work-ing lives. At times, staff in the service simply did not agree with what the users wanted. The question of when it is appropriate and acceptable for staff to reject or over-ride users' suggestions is an im-portant tension which we consider in more detail in Chapter 7.

Inevitably, if a consultation is inclusive, a redesign event will gen-erate a diversity of views about the appropriate solution to any problem – and at times overt conflict between users may emerge. Disagreement can be daunting to deal with, though consensus-building techniques such as the nominal group method can offer a systematic and equitable way of achieving a middle ground.[11]

We found that even when staff were broadly in favour of change, translating user suggestions into a service improvement solution was not always a straightforward process. For example, user feed-back may say 'the receptionist was rude'. This may reflect a gen-uine training need in the reception staff for customer care skills, but it may also reflect the users' anxiety about the service more generally, articulated as a personal criticism of a receptionist but for which a more appropriate solution would be a much more general redesign of the accessibility and friendliness of the clinic. By step-ping outside of the direct user experience we observed that there were many complex factors that contributed to what appeared to be a specific piece of feedback. We learnt that we needed to care-fully contextualise user feedback and that effective 'solutions' often needed to address multiple elements and levels of the service.

Challenge 8: Achieving closure

On one hand, quality improvement (and hence, user involvement in quality improvement) is an ongoing, never-ending issue for any healthcare service. On the other hand, particular sub-projects ad-dressing particular aspects of the service usually have a beginning, a main phase, and an ending – and the time-limited nature of an initiative can focus goals to be set and short-term targets for par-ticular outputs met. This can potentially create confusion amongst users about what their current relationship with the service is. We found that there are no hard and fast rules here, but that sensitivity to what users and staff may be feeling, and to the wider internal and external pressures on the service is important.

In some cases achieving closure on a sub-project, especially when user involvement had been short-term and relatively limited, was as simple as thanking everyone for their participation, undertaking to let people know the outcome, and addressing practicalities such as meeting travel expenses and one-off payments. In other cases, follow-through was necessary to take forward suggestions (for example, a sub-group might be formed to provide ongoing feedback on a particular initiative, or a further event might be organised to feed back fleshed-out plans in a more structured and consultative way).

Two further issues sometimes arose, however. The first was how to sustain fresh and appropriate engagement over time (and avoid the problem of a cohort of 'usual suspects' who expected to be reinvited for every new user involvement event). We found that the appropriate intensity and length of user involvement varied with the task. Sometimes, as in the mystery shopper project, involvement of a particular group of individuals matured and changed over time, and the experienced users themselves took on the task of bringing in 'new blood'. At other times, awkward moments occurred when a user who had taken on a 'professional patient' role was told that someone other than them was needed for a particular task or project – usually because staff felt that this person was no longer speaking for 'ordinary' patients. This clearly raises questions about power relations in the project (who should be allowed to say that a particular user is 'no longer needed', and why?) which are discussed further in Chapter 7.

The second was how to disengage sensitively after users had been involved in a particularly intensive redesign effort, perhaps following an adverse experience in the service by themselves or others. In some such cases, the needs of the participants as patients may have to be considered – for example by encouraging or helping them to raise any unresolved issues with the clinician responsible for their care.

One way of achieving closure in some of the MI sub-projects was a 'ceremonial event' in which the service users who had contributed to a redesign effort participated in the launch of a new service or a celebration of its success. Some examples of this are covered in Chapter 5.

Finally, linking with third-sector organisations and groupings such as the Kidney Patient Association or stroke service user networks can be a good way for users to shift their focus and efforts (and recharge their batteries!) after helping with a particular time-limited project.

Summary: Ten tips for successful co-design

1 When identifying potential users to be involved in an initiative, think carefully what sort of users to ask and what each might contribute. Different recruitment strategies may be needed for different groups and sub-groups. Some groups are likely to remain excluded unless you specifically seek to identify and recruit them.

2 'Taster' experiences of user involvement (such as ad hoc waiting room discussions) may introduce users to the idea of participation.

3 Try to view the user involvement experience in your project through the eyes of a user, and address the 'what's in it for me?' question. Make involvement easy, flexible and fulfilling. In particular, make it clear to people what *they* can contribute to a particular focused aspect of service improvement.

4 Address practicalities such as travel, expenses, refreshments and reimbursement. These can be extremely important, especially for low-income participants and attention to such issues encourages diverse participation.

5 In a preparation phase, make sure all participants (users and staff) are clear about what is required of them and what it is possible to change.

6 Make your expectations clear and get agreement on these – for example in relation to attendance, timekeeping, and the nature and standard of any written input. Provide training and support if the last of these is needed.

7 In the problem identification phase, create a safe and supportive environment to allow honest, constructive criticism of existing services.

8 In the solution generation phase, support imaginative thinking – perhaps by using examples from services elsewhere or even outside healthcare.

9 When selecting solutions and planning changes, anticipate conflicts between different participants and also between what has been suggested and what is practically possible. Good facilitation is critical and there may be a place for formal consensus-building techniques.

10 After a time-limited project, consider how to achieve closure. If users' involvement has been intensive and/or addressed sensitive issues, users may need further support.

References

1. Bate SP, Robert G. *Bringing User Experience to Healthcare Improvement.* Oxford: Radcliffe; 2007.
2. Bate P, Robert G. Toward more user-centric OD: lessons from the field of experience-based design and a case study. *J Appl Behav Sci* 2007; 43(1):41–66.
3. van Staa A, Jedeloo S, Latour J, Trappenburg MJ. Exciting but exhausting: experiences with participatory research with chronically ill adolescents. *Health Expect* 2010; 13(1):95–107.
4. Iliffe S, Manthorpe J, Drennan V, Goodman C, Warner J. The EVIDEM programme: a test for primary care research in London? *Lond J Prim Care* 2008; 1(1):69–73.
5. Needham C. Realising the potential of co-production: negotiating improvements in public services. *Soc Policy Soc* 2008; 7(2):221–231.
6. Baraitser P, Pearce V, Blake G, Collander-Brown K, Ridley A. Involving service users in sexual health service development. *J Fam Plann Reprod Health Care* 2005; 31:281–284.
7. Baraitser P, Pearce V, Walsh N, Cooper R, Brown KC, Holmes J et al. Look who's taking notes in your clinic: mystery shoppers as evaluators in sexual health services. *Health Expect* 2008; 11(1):54–62.
8. Anonymous. *Mystery Shopping in Sexual Health: A Toolkit for Delivery.* Downloadable from http://www.gsttcharity.org.uk/pdfs/mystery.pdf. London: Modernisation Initiative; 2008.
9. Anonymous. *Improving Services by Involving Patients, Carers and Staff: A Step by Step Guide to Organising Whole-system Service Improvement Events.* London: Modernisation Initiative; 2007.
10. Boynton PM, Wood GW, Greenhalgh T. A hands on guide to questionnaire research part three: reaching beyond the white middle classes. *BMJ* 2004; 328(7453):1433–1436.
11. Elwyn G, Greenhalgh T, Macfarlane F. *Groups – A Hands-on Guide to Small Group Work in Education, Management and Research.* Oxford: Radcliffe; 2000.

CHAPTER 4

Patients as teachers and mentors

Gaynor Smith[1], Jane Hughes[2] & Trisha Greenhalgh[3]
[1]End of Life Care, Guys and St Thomas' Modernisation Initiative, London, UK
[2]City University, London, UK
[3]Queen Mary, University of London, London, UK

As Chapter 2 showed, it is widely accepted in both academic and policy circles that patients and carers bring a special type of expertise to a service from which others (clinical staff, managers and other service users) may learn.[1–9] In this chapter, we offer two very different examples of patients as teachers and mentors. The first is an account of how people who had had strokes and their carers became involved in the education of staff, and the second describes a peer support initiative for patients and carers in the kidney service.

Example 1: Learning from people living with stroke

The first phase of this work adopted a model known as 'patients as teachers' that had been used successfully in other services.[3] A member of the stroke modernisation initiative (MI) staff had previous experience of using this approach. The patients as teachers model aims to:

- Identify issues that matter to service users
- Develop user defined good practice guidance
- Provide opportunities for service users to train clinicians
- Identify mutually agreed areas for service development with clearly defined outcomes

---

User Involvement in Health Care, 1st edition. Edited by Trisha Greenhalgh, Charlotte Humphrey and Fran Woodard. © 2011 Blackwell Publishing Ltd.

People who were willing to share their experiences of stroke were invited to take part in facilitated focus groups. Facilitators also organised meetings with members of several stroke support groups. In total, more than 40 people took part in these group discussions, which ensured diversity of experience. Participants were encouraged to talk about what had happened to them and the services they had received; they were asked what had worked well or, if they pointed out shortcomings, what would have constituted good care. From this broad range of experiences and views, project staff distilled the issues that mattered to service users and these became a booklet of good practice guidance to be used in training local health and social care staff. Additionally, film footage of some groups and individuals telling their stories provided material for a DVD to accompany and illustrate the points made in the booklet.

A group of people living with stroke continued their involvement in the project by co-presenting training sessions for staff in stroke units, primary care and social services. At some training sessions, the DVD was shown and several of the service users who appeared in it acted as an 'expert panel', responding to questions and contributing to discussion. Participating staff used the training sessions to review their professional practice and to identify areas for local service development.

Developing the good practice guidance stimulated further initiatives to improve services for people living with stroke and some of the service users who had taken part in the discussion groups continued their engagement with the work.

At the end of the first phase of this initiative, the stroke service users and carers who had been involved were invited to a meeting to talk about taking the work further. In the course of the project, people had got to know each other and had become increasingly confident about talking about their strokes. Some of them joined a group to collaborate to design and plan 'raising awareness' events in primary care for professionals and patients to hear about and discuss the experience of stroke. The events were informal, with service users taking an active role and participating in an 'expert panel' to answer questions.

This was seen by both service users and primary care staff as an effective way of getting all stakeholders to work together, increasing their understanding of what it is like to live with stroke, and encouraging debate about how to improve services. After two planned events had been held, several of the involved service users went to their own general practices (GP) and tried to persuade them to organise a raising awareness event. This was not easy – one participant described how they had '*harassed and harassed*' to try to engage their own GP. Eventually two practices did so, and the events were perceived as highly successful – in particular, attendance was high and the practice was described as '*hugely surprised*'. Some of the patients who attended the events became involved in the work of the project and several went on to join other local and national initiatives for people living with stroke.

The 'patients as teachers' approach drew on users' stroke experiences in a specific way – to construct patient narratives for the purpose of teaching staff. The idea was to get across the essence of which issues matter to patients, how and why – similar in some ways to distilling 'good practice guidance', but this was created by educators and took the form of stories about the patient's care. In this approach, narratives are seen to introduce an 'affective understanding' rather than merely the 'cognitive response' that is more usual in professional discourse.[10, 11]

The patient perspective, captured in narratives, was seen as a very powerful way of challenging professionals' views about the quality of services and how services are delivered to patients. The medium of film conveyed a sense of authority to the user, especially if the user was present in the flesh for a subsequent question and answer session. The narrative approach seemed to focus staff on thinking about their own position in the organisation, enabling them to consider how care could be improved. Some staff felt that they could 'see themselves through the patient's eyes'. But the impact of stories on staff was not predictable or consistent – different staff had very different responses, and indeed the variability in response sometimes sparked fruitful discussion. Many staff commented that the authentic patient voice had a powerful impact in discussions, which was hard to ignore or dismiss.

> *I think it's partly about seeing them out of their role as anonymous patients. They are an expert patient and that's given some credibility in the context of training, which seems to affect how people listen to what they say, both professionals and other service users. Also it humanises, it's actually quite difficult to dismiss what they're saying because they come over as human, not just a patient who has had a stroke. And the professionals have been appreciative of patients giving up their time to come and talk to the teams.* (Doctor, stroke services)

The stroke project team developed a DVD and website *'Learning from People who have had Strokes'*, available as a free download from http://www.gsttcharity.org.uk/grants/results_mistroke.html#x1.

Example 2: Peer support in the kidney service

The idea of developing peer support grew out of early consultation meetings with kidney patients and their families, who emphasised the value of talking to other patients, which often happened informally in outpatient clinics and on the hospital wards. It was also clear to MI project staff that participants at 'whole system events' (see Chapter 3) enjoyed meeting others who were 'in the same boat', although this had not been the primary reason for organising the events. Professionals from kidney services at the two hospital trusts working with the project were also interested in exploring the value of a more formalised approach to enabling patients to share experiences.

The first step was to be clear about what was being offered. There is no single definition of peer support and it has similarities with, as well as important differences from, other ways of providing information and support such as befriending, buddying, peer education and peer mentoring.[12, 13] Project staff did some background research and presented the findings to a meeting of service users and carers to find out what they wanted. A broad consensus was established: peer support should be short-term and complement care provided by professionals; it should be provided by volunteer patients who had received training, and it should be accessed through a link nurse, who would match patient and peer supporter. Both patients and staff felt that suitably trained peer supporters could use their experience of living with kidney disease to help others, particularly patients who were about to begin treatment.

The peer support service model was formally defined as:[14]

- An additional service available to patients if they want it
- Complementary to care and education by professionals
- Provided by volunteer patients who have received training and preparation for the role of peer supporter
- A single meeting or telephone conversation offering short-term support, rather than an attempt to establish a longer term relationship or 'befriending'

- Managed by link nurses, who match each patient with a suitable peer supporter
- Accessed by a patient contacting the link nurse directly or being referred by a clinician

A steering group including service users and clinicians was formed to implement peer support. Volunteers were recruited and they helped to refine ideas and plans, including the content and organisation of the training. The first group of peer supporters worked with the link nurses to finalise the practical details of how peer support would be delivered; they also provided feedback on their training that was used to improve subsequent courses. The link nurses provided support for the peer supporters, for example talking through issues raised in the training and dealing with any issues that arose in their discussions with patients.

Referrals for peer support from the clinical kidney services were very low initially, which created some dissatisfaction among the cadre of trained peer supporters who were eager to 'get going'. Some exploratory interviews suggested that many clinicians either did not 'believe in' peer support or did not understand how to refer patients to the service. As a result of this feedback, changes were made to the way peer support was presented to clinicians and a publicity campaign launched to encourage patients to contact the link nurses directly. Eventually a steady flow of referrals was achieved. It was discovered that peer supporters with certain types of treatment experience were called on more frequently than others.

Evaluation confirmed that patients who had spoken to a peer supporter felt it had helped them in variety of ways, notably by providing reassurance, building confidence, giving access to information which 'the doctors wouldn't know', and helping them make a personal decision about treatment (for example, whether haemodialysis or peritoneal dialysis would suit them better).[14]

Peer support had originally been conceptualised as providing hands-on information and support for patients who were having difficulty making treatment decisions. As experience accumulated, however, it became apparent that this model could be of more general value. At the time of writing, all patients in participating kidney services are encouraged to access peer support whenever they feel they need it (Figure 4.1).

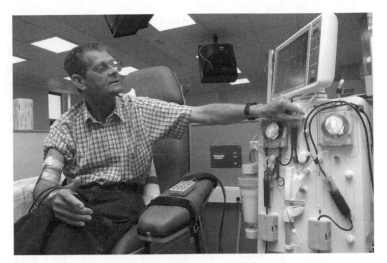

Figure 4.1 Patient learning to self-manage on dialysis.

Challenge 1: Recognising where the expertise lies

Despite much encouragement at policy level, the idea of patients as teachers and mentors is profoundly challenging to the conventional view of the patient role. There is a risk that initiatives may pay lip-service to the rhetoric of the 'expert' patient while still constructing the patient in what is fundamentally a passive, ignorant and inactive role. At one end of the spectrum, service users may be invited to provide first hand experience for the benefit of students but still be treated by staff as exhibits of symptomatologies who may be probed and questioned, but who have no voice in determining the direction of education or training.[2] One user who subsequently became a peer supporter described how she had been inspired to get involved after seeing a fellow patient being 'wheeled in' and told to speak on cue:

> *I remember going to one of those renal education programmes – you have to do that to get onto the transplant list. A woman came on – the patient always comes on last. The least significant person, the bottom of the heap. A carefully selected patient and organised not to say too much, to be, more than anything, positive. . . .* (Kidney patient, member of steering group for patient involvement work)

At the other end of the spectrum, there are many excellent examples in the literature of groups of service users who have been commissioned to devise, deliver and assess entire training courses or modules.[1] In between are models of partnership in which service users and staff work together. Depending on the specific approach taken, there is a risk of 'dilution' or compromise of user perspectives or of reflecting a rather marginal and tokenistic involvement of service users, perhaps 'slotting them in' to an existing curriculum and style of teaching. Lack of confidence and experience on both sides, and/or lack of time and resources, will factor against the more radical and imaginative models.

The two examples given in this chapter both describe initiatives where user involvement was sought from the outset and the project was deemed a success. It is worth mentioning briefly an initiative in the kidney MI where the user's expertise was *not* initially sought because patient expertise was not identified as key. A training module in communication skills for clinical staff was commissioned as a result of a user consultation, but the staff training did not initially have any direct service user involvement. The module was received with mixed views. At about the same time, staff discovered that a kidney patient had written a play about waiting for a transplant and asked him to write some scenarios of clinician and patient consultations in which there are communication difficulties. This patient worked with a member of staff to write a number of scenarios that were performed by actors at several events. These were highly effective in getting service users and staff to talk about issues from a patient's perspective. The scenarios were later filmed so they could be used more regularly in staff training.

Challenge 2: Clarifying roles and responsibilities

A recurring theme in our experience of involving patients and carers in teaching/mentoring roles, which is also described in the wider literature, is the need to be clear about who is doing what.[1-6] Patients and carers do not want to replace professionals. Theirs is a very different type of expertise built on experiential, embodied knowledge. One of the commonest concerns expressed by users was the need for reliable back up from designated professionals (most commonly nurses), to whom they could refer any problem which they themselves felt unqualified to deal with. Hopes were sometimes expressed by enthusiastic health professionals or managers that patient mentors might *replace* clinical staff (thereby saving money); such hopes were usually based on a naïve model of how the division of labour would play out between users and professionals.

In general, we found that whilst professionals tended to need considerable clarification of roles and responsibilities in the peer support project, patients did not. They knew that they were getting something quite different from other patients than they were getting from professional staff, and they rarely seemed to be confused about the roles and responsibilities. Peer supporters saw their role as conveying the lived experience of the different management options and explaining key points in lay terms, not as providing sophisticated medical or technical expertise.

A doctor is a doctor . . . they talk in a different tone than a normal person would. It takes an average person, someone from the public who is going through the same problem as you, to know where you're coming from. Even though doctors are human, they talk in a different code. . . . the doctors say this has happened to you, the percentage is that, you need to take this for your bones . . . You can't absorb all that stuff. It takes time. I'm not the sharpest chisel in the box and it took a long time to get that marinated into me. . . . I had to learn it myself. Listening to a doctor is like gobbledegook, I couldn't understand it, I had to take it in myself.

because a doctor, for all the information they know, they haven't actually lived it themselves

. . . you want to know how it's going to affect you and what you're going to do. And that's all that matters. The person on the street who's got the disease, who's coping with the same problem as you, he knows how to deal with it and he can tell you how to deal with it. (Kidney patients reflecting on experience of peer support)

Challenge 3: Overcoming staff resistance

Professionals who had not previously been 'taught' by patients were often wary of the new service model. Some were concerned about implicit power shifts and their own vulnerability to criticism or exposure. In our experience, this negativity tended to attenuate as staff experienced the positive benefits of patients as teachers.

> *there can be a fear that they're going to get criticised. And mostly that doesn't happen. They realise there's a great overlap in what's important to them. And it can surprise professionals and reassure them and quite often they get a lot of positive feedback from service users, which is very affirming and creates a lot of energy.* (Service improvement facilitator)

Similarly, clinicians who had no experience with service users as peer supporters sometimes took several months to start referring patients to the scheme. In the peer support example, most staff resistance did not appear to be about 'power' issues but stemmed from a lack of understanding of what peer support was for and how it might add value. In addition, referring to the organised peer support service was an additional step in staff routines, involving (for example) an extra phone call. Most commonly, apparent resistance to the scheme was linked to the attitude 'we're doing it already' – meaning, in an ad hoc and sometimes inappropriate way, by asking a patient who happened to be on the dialysis unit or in the clinic to talk to the individual who was about to start a similar form of treatment. A crucial step was to make the service open for patients to request a peer support link themselves without going through a clinician.[14]

We found that one way of overcoming staff resistance was including positive messages about users as teachers or mentors within other aspects of staff training, rather than seeing this work as a freestanding and isolated project that was not mentioned elsewhere in the curriculum.

Challenge 4: Supporting users in their teaching/mentoring role

As Manthorpe has shown in relation to the involvement of carers in social work education, there are both benefits and risks associated with presenting 'real life' experience in an effort to enlighten and train professionals.[15] Not only are users expected to reveal personal and potentially stigmatising information to people who are not directly involved in their own care, there is also the risk of stereotyping. And standing up in front of a group of health professionals (some of whom may be silently challenging one's 'expertise') can be daunting.

We found that in general, service users tended to grow in confidence and became very passionate about what they were trying to achieve. In some cases, users valued opportunities to practise and build confidence in informal settings prior to the official teaching sessions. We also found an unexpected benefit in terms of increased confidence generally:

> *A lot of people developed their confidence to do things that initially they wouldn't have done. . . . we've had people getting up and talking in front of groups and at conferences. For some people it was about getting up there despite their communication difficulty and having a go anyway . . . some of them would say it's helped improve their communication. Some have gained confidence to get paid work. Others have made friends as a result of taking part.* (Service improvement facilitator)

In the kidney peer support example, one initial problem was that having volunteered to be a peer supporter, some people did not get called upon by the service because of the low initial referral rate. The link nurse role was vital to managing relationships and ensuring that peer supporters were kept 'on board' at this time. Link nurses also provided a crucial facility for peer supporters to talk through issues raised (e.g. confidentiality).

Challenge 5: Practicalities

Many of the practical issues relating to user involvement in teaching and mentoring have already been covered in the previous chapter. They include the need for an administrative infrastructure (especially a point of contact and a database of people who are willing to be approached), the questions of how to fund the service and whether and how to remunerate users, the need to prepare users for their role and support them in that role and the operational challenges of group work. In addition, statutory checks (e.g. Criminal Records Bureau) had to be completed before users were allowed to provide a formal support service to other users. The 'administrative' issues in peer support also included the ability to match a new patient with a suitable peer supporter, which required considerable experience and insight from the link nurse about how the interpersonal relationship would play out – something that could probably not have been done by a non-clinician lacking knowledge of the particular patients.

The kidney MI project published an extensive guide to such practicalities which is downloadable in full text (http://www.gsttcharity. org.uk/pdfs/whitecoat.pdf).[14] Most of these challenges have also been described by others in similar and contrasting projects to involve users in teaching or mentoring.[1–3,10,12,15,16]

Summary: Ten tips for involving service users in teaching or mentoring

1 Involve users from the outset when designing a new teaching or mentoring programme.

2 Be absolutely clear about what service users are 'experts' in and what their role would be in any particular initiative.

3 Acknowledge that the user as 'expert' is profoundly challenging to traditional views on the patient or carer role, hence expect that there may be resistance from many staff.

4 Prepare and train staff so that they understand what users are and are not expected to do, and what their own role in the initiative will be. Manage any expectations or fears that users might replace professionals.

5 Ensure that the user experience has central importance in the teaching or mentoring initiative – for example by placing particular value on first-person narratives told without interruption or editing by professionals.

6 Recognise that there will be a tendency to slip into tokenistic (and even voyeuristic) involvement of patients and carers within conventional teaching programmes. Take steps to ensure that the user voice is heard and respected whenever users are said to be 'involved'.

7 Provide adequate administrative support, especially a point of contact and a searchable database of potential contributors.

8 Provide adequate clinical support for patient mentors – preferably a 'hot line' to a nurse or equivalent professional.

9 Help users build their confidence – for example by offering opportunities for informal 'dry run' sessions or linking with other users in a similar role.

10 Address practical issues such as expenses and remuneration.

References

1. Repper J, Breeze J. User and carer involvement in the training and education of health professionals: a review of the literature. *Int J Nurs Stud* 2007; 44(3):511–519.
2. Townend M, Tew J, Grant A, Repper J. Involvement of service users in education and training: A review of the literature and exploration of the implications for the education and training of psychological therapists. *J Ment Health* 2008; 17(1):65–78.
3. Wykurz G, Kelly D. Developing the role of patients as teachers: literature review. *BMJ* 2002; 325(7368):818–821.
4. Peck E, Barker I. Users as partners in mental health – ten years of experience. *J Interprof Care* 1997; 11:269–277.
5. Florin D, Dixon J. Public involvement in health care. *BMJ* 2004; 328:159–161.
6. Bate SP, Robert G. *Bringing User Experience to Healthcare Improvement*. Oxford: Radcliffe; 2007.
7. Tew J, Gell C, Foster S. *Learning from Experience. Involving Service Users and Carers in Mental Health Education and Training*. York: Higher Education Academy, NIMHE, Trent Workforce Development Confederation; 2004.
8. Barnes D, Carpenter J, Bailey D. Partnerships with service users in interprofessional education for community mental health: a case study. *J Interprof Care* 2000; 14(2):189–200.
9. Reynolds J, Read J. Opening minds: user involvement in the production of learning materials on mental health and distress. *Soc Work Educ* 1999; 18(4):417–431.
10. Blickem C, Priyadharshini E. Patient Narratives: the potential for "patient-centred" interprofessional learning? *J Interprof Care* 2007; 21(6):619–632.
11. Ziebland S, Herxheimer A. How patients' experiences contribute to decision making: illustrations from DIPEx (personal experiences of health and illness). *J Nurs Manag* 2008; 16(4):433–439.
12. Dennis CL. Peer support within a health care context: a concept analysis. *Int J Nurs Stud* 2003; 40(3):321–332.
13. World Health Organization. Peer support programmes in diabetes: Report of a WHO consultation 5–7 November 2007. Geneva: WHO; 2008.
14. Hughes J, Wood E, Cox S, Silas L, Smith G. 'No white coat between us'. *Developing Peer Support Services for Kidney Patients*. London: Modernisation Initiative; 2008. Available at http://www.gsttcharity.org.uk/pdfs/whitecoat.pdf.
15. Manthorpe J. Developing carers' contributions to social work training. *Soc Work Educ* 2000; 19(1):19–27.
16. Gupta A, Blewett J. Involving service users in social work training on the reality of family poverty: a case study of a collaborative project. *Soc Work Educ* 2008; 27(5):459–473.

CHAPTER 5

Co-producing information

Jane Hughes[1], Gaynor Smith[2] & Trisha Greenhalgh[3]
[1]City University, London, UK
[2]End of Life Care, Guys and St Thomas' Modernisation Initiative, London, UK
[3]Queen Mary, University of London, London, UK

All three projects in the modernisation initiative (MI) found that service users identified the quality and availability of information as a significant area for improvement. All the projects explored and addressed this in partnership with users. In the wider literature, many authors have written on the poor quality of information available to patients and carers on the nature of their condition, possible treatment options, risks and benefits of different options, and the nature of services and how to access them.[1–4] These reports suggest that there is often no shortage of information but that it is typically poorly and inconsistently presented and inadequately personalised (i.e. it does not include the particular things that patients want to know).

Furthermore, professionals in general do not proactively provide information to patients; there is little co-ordination between information providers across sectoral or organisational boundaries, and services are often characterised by a lack of 'signposting'. As a report from the Picker Institute put it in 2006: *'many patient information leaflets and websites do not provide sufficiently accurate and detailed information to assist patients in making decisions about their healthcare'*.[1]

The same authors published a report via the World Health Organisation in 2008 arguing that when making decisions about care, patients need information and education to help them decide between different treatment options and support self-management.[5]

User Involvement in Health Care, 1st edition. Edited by Trisha Greenhalgh, Charlotte Humphrey and Fran Woodard. © 2011 Blackwell Publishing Ltd.

The challenge is not just about providing high-quality information resources; a coherent strategy is needed to inform and empower patients, including ensuring that healthcare staff have good communication skills and are encouraging patients to take an active role in their own care.

Marshall et al. showed in 2006 that for service users (and perhaps providers too) who had little or no experience of working together to improve services, information provided a focus for engagement that was tangible, and perceived as legitimate and uncontentious.[6] Users felt they needed access to better information about services to redress the power imbalance with providers. Thus, the provision of information can potentially be a catalyst for engaging service users.

Below, we describe four contrasting examples of involving users in producing (or co-producing) information for other service users. Our experience across the three MI projects suggests that producing information is a practical and safe way for patients and carers to begin their involvement in service transformation. The commitment is usually fairly well defined and focused on a tangible product. Each of the examples below raises some challenges however, which are discussed in the later parts of this chapter.

Example 1: Co-producing DVDs for kidney patients

The kidney MI project produced a number of DVDs and booklets for patients. The first of these was a DVD about living donor transplant which was designed by professionals to provide patients with the information it was considered they needed to know. This DVD was seen as a positive start but criticised for using a 'talking heads' (consultants speaking to camera) format and failing to address the questions patients really wanted answered.

The second DVD came out of discussion at 'Dialysis Choices', a group of professionals and patients set up with a view to improving all aspects of dialysis services. This group had identified a gap in information about how patients manage their own dialysis. There was (at the time) no readily available resource which explained how patients doing their own dialysis could fit their treatment into their lives and maintain independence. A project worker (who had a nursing background) was given the brief to produce a DVD. She interviewed 25 self-caring patients to capture their perspectives and establish the issues that needed to be included.

The patients who agreed to be filmed decided how they wanted their lives to be portrayed. They devised a standard set of questions about life on dialysis and the film was edited to highlight particular aspects of different types of treatment. At all stages in production, the project worker checked the content of the DVD with the patients who were featured and with a separate patient information panel to ensure it was easy to understand and acceptable in tone and emphasis. Clinicians were also consulted. It was a long process and fraught with disagreement, but patients had the final say.

The effort that went into developing '*Living Life to the Full on Dialysis*' was considered worthwhile: this second DVD was acknowledged to have broken new ground as a resource for kidney patients and it was enthusiastically received by patients and clinicians alike (Figure 5.1).

Building on this success, a similar approach was taken to developing another DVD to provide more comprehensive clinical information about kidney disease and the various treatments available. Patients, carers and clinicians who took part in an event to discuss provision for educating patients before they started treatment had identified a range of issues including the appropriateness of information available and how it was delivered. To supplement their feedback, a project worker decided to interview a cross section of patients who were at an early stage in treatment to find out what information they had received, what they had found useful and what else they wanted. This offered some surprising insights: many people were resistant to receiving information, for emotional or cultural reasons, carers often got more out of the information provided than patients, and levels of health and information literacy were an issue.

The third DVD and booklet '*Your Kidneys, Your Choice*' was developed with these points in mind. It was modelled on a DVD from Belgium and although clinicians decided what should be covered, the script was written jointly by a clinician and a patient who was a professional scriptwriter. Clinical accuracy of the information was paramount, but the text was reviewed by a patient information panel to check their understanding and resolve any disagreements about wording. Images and simple diagrams were also extensively used to show how treatments worked, and these were strongly influenced by consultation sessions with patients, which determined how the diagrams should look and how much detail to include, before they were given to a designer. The second part of the DVD showed patients talking about the practicalities of

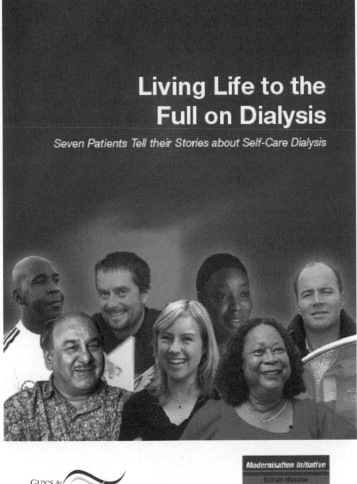

Figure 5.1 Book '*Living Life to the Full on Dialysis*' written by users and staff.

various forms of treatment and how these fitted into their lives. Service users were involved throughout production: the patient information panel commented on the booklet and DVD at different stages of development and a steering group including clinicians and patients oversaw the whole process.

Overall, participants in the kidney MI project felt that the involvement of service users in the production of these DVDs had become both more sophisticated and more effective as the project developed and they learnt lessons from both the strengths and limitations of their previous efforts. Clinicians in particular spoke positively about both the process of making the DVD with patients and the impact of the DVD on their own learning and attitudes. For example:

> *When we saw the DVD, we saw patients in another light, as real people living their lives...* (Doctor, kidney services)
>
> *The insight I got from him, it was a very different situation ... I found it affected my thinking a lot, personally and professionally, but then I spent many days working with him. And I found that hugely useful on a personal level and in terms of what we produced. I enjoyed it.* (Nurse who worked with the patient on scripting the DVD)

Example 2: A small-scale project to develop accessible menus for stroke patients

The MI stroke team invited groups of people living with stroke (patients and their carers) to discuss their experiences of services. One of the problems identified was that patients with aphasia had difficulty making their needs known to hospital staff. Patients had typically been asked to order their food from the menus that were distributed in the ward each day, which required them to read small-font print and tick boxes to make their choices. The patients were unable to choose from the menus because their recent stroke had affected their ability to read or understand the printed information. They found this upsetting, particularly since food was one of the few pleasures in life at that difficult time. A typical comment was *'no-one asked me if I could read and I got food I didn't want'*.

A working group comprising former stroke patients, a speech and language therapist, catering staff and a photographer set out to develop 'accessible menus' and picture boards for the stroke wards. The menus had photographs of the meals and an accompanying image to make clear what the meal contained. For example, chicken pie would have a photograph of a piece of pie as well as an image of a chicken. The menus were piloted with the group and on the wards, and quickly entered regular use. Patients unable to find the words to ask for help could use the picture boards to communicate their needs.

This example shows that user involvement in the production of information can be very effective in small-scale projects, and that the starting point for successful information projects is often a candid assessment of the user experience.

Example 3: Strategic-level involvement of stroke patients in developing an information strategy

In a much larger initiative in the stroke MI, about 60 people living with stroke took part in two 'Join in' events to talk about their experiences of stroke and discuss their ideas for improving stroke information and support. They wanted timely access to appropriate information about the nature of stroke, the range of services available locally and the opportunities available for support and rehabilitation. Following this consultation, an advisory group of 14 members was formed (the Stroke Information Advisory Group, SIAG), on which were represented service users, carers, and health and social care professionals.

The SIAG mapped in some detail service users' experience of receiving stroke information, working in small groups to talk about their patient journey, what information they had needed at each point, the most appropriate format and what it felt like to receive information (or not). This material was collated into the Stroke Information Pathway, based on work on patient information pathways pioneered in cancer services, to provide a record of patient-defined information needs that could be used as a benchmark for assessing current information provision and to identify examples of good practice, as well as gaps and deficiencies.

The group found that there was a great deal of information available for people living with stroke, although there were also some notable gaps which the SIAG took steps to fill. The main issue however was that information was inaccessible or not given to people at the right time. Better 'signposting' was considered to be the solution. To this end, the group developed a stroke patient handbook, a 'filofax'-type patient held record for all patients, with sections covering the whole pathway of care, references to relevant information at each stage and questions that patients may wish to ask professionals. To fill gaps in information, the group developed resources including ward leaflets and booklets, pictorial hospital menus and a transient ischaemic attack (TIA) handbook (a personalised information resource about TIA and stroke prevention).

A number of younger service users who had come to meetings organised by the MI identified that there were no resources for people living with stroke who were parents of school age or younger children. They formed a group and worked on the production of a DVD and a book, 'Having a Stroke, Being a Parent – A Guide for Parents with Stroke and Aphasia and their Families' based on their experiences. The aim of these was to provide ideas, inspiration and support for parents who had sustained stroke and/or aphasia. The DVD was sponsored by 'Connect', the national communication disability network, with an advisory group of eight service users.

The DVD presented real-life experiences, and the people featured reflected the diversity of parents living with stroke in terms of gender, ethnicity, sexual orientation and level of disability. It also presented a child's perspective. The success of the DVD cannot be measured by the number of copies sold because its target audience is relatively small. However, the positive response, nationally and locally, indicated that it had met the aim of addressing their particular circumstances and needs. The DVD is available from Connect (http://www.ukconnect.org/).

Example 4: Developing and improving sexual health information

The users of the sexual health service in this project were characterised by wide ethnic and social diversity, variable levels of health literacy and intermittent contact with the service. Many were young and had had limited contact with health services for any purpose. Epidemiological data collected by the genito-urinary and gynaecology services suggested that the people presenting to the service with sexually transmitted infections or unwanted pregnancies represented only the tip of an iceberg of unmet need in the wider community – in other words, most people stayed away from the service either because they did not know or care about it or because they were frightened of seeking care. 'Sexual health' includes a vast range of conditions in people representing different sexual orientations. All these factors combined to pose a major challenge for the team who sought to produce a comprehensive, accessible set of information for all users and potential users of the service.

The sexual health MI decided to begin with a series of focus groups to develop materials to promote low cost condoms to 18–24-year-olds in a particular area of South London with high levels of social deprivation. An earlier needs assessment had shown that people seemed to be willing to buy condoms. Focus groups were organised opportunistically where young people gathered, for example at youth groups, and participants were asked to look at the campaign materials and comment on them. Other young people using a health information library were also interviewed individually about their reactions to the images and text. The campaign was successful insofar as condom sales locally increased significantly after it.

Another campaign was to increase awareness amongst young people of a local pharmacy-based service for sexual health information and services, particularly Chlamydia testing. Leaflets and posters had been designed, but there were concerns about whether they got the messages across to all target groups in the population. Mystery shoppers (see Chapter 3) evaluated the information in pharmacies, and the first time round made many negative comments.

Before running the campaign again, the materials were changed and tested with two further focus groups. One was held at a centre where asylum seekers and refugees met regularly. The other was advertised to young people who used sexual health services. Participants were given a £10 voucher for participating in the groups. Both groups included about 10 people and were run by an experienced facilitator. Participants wanted the materials to emphasise more clearly that this was a free service; they also suggested that messages should be simpler and more straightforward and the posters should be displayed more prominently in the pharmacies. The leaflets and posters were amended accordingly.

The mystery shoppers were again asked to provide feedback on how the materials were used in the pharmacies. This time, before their visits, the mystery shoppers were briefed about the campaign and what could be expected from participating community pharmacies, bearing in mind that they are small businesses with limited time and space. The mystery shopper reports were more positive and their criticisms welcomed as constructive and helpful by the pharmacists.

Before running the campaign a third time, more focus groups were held with different groups and further changes made. The young people wanted even simpler, shorter messages and the materials were redesigned. Feedback from service users was more positive than previously. The 30 participating community pharmacists were surveyed for their views. They thought the campaign materials had improved: they were easier for customers to understand, especially that it was a free service, which helped them to promote the services. Many still had the posters on display and reported that customers were asking for sexual health advice.

This relatively low cost campaign was considered by participants to have been effective and the value of involving service users in developing materials was judged by service managers to have been well worth the effort of running the focus groups and organising the mystery shopper evaluation. A similar approach was subsequently used to improve a leaflet about termination of pregnancy, which had initially been produced without any service user input. Five focus groups, each with ten women and independently facilitated, reviewed the content of the leaflet. Clear recommendations for improvement were acted on and the leaflet was reprinted and positively received.

All these examples raise important challenges facing those who seek to co-produce information with service users.

Challenge 1: Making the user experience the starting point

A strong thread running through all the MI work was users' experience as a way into improving service quality. Initiatives to develop information and education tended to use a biographical approach: as the above examples show, real patients were featured in information materials (posters, booklets, DVDs) and took part in delivering information and (as described in Chapter 4) face to face training for health professionals.

As the last example above shows, information materials designed without user input often had to be redesigned to make them meaningful and engaging to users. One of the major learning points from the MI was that when the 'unedited' user experience was the starting point, a change initiative seemed to have an unparalleled sense of authenticity, importance and immediacy. On the contrary, when the user experience was inserted tokenistically or as a footnote to an otherwise professionally led strategy, the project had (in the words of one project lead) less 'buzz and energy' and less impact.

Challenge 2: Capturing stories

Stories are a natural tool for learning, but when used in information materials, they have to be elicited, selected, shortened, and illustrated (see the Patient Voices website, www.patientvoices. org.uk, for more details on these 'storywork' tasks and worked examples of stories edited and illustrated in collaboration with patients). The MI developed different ways of capturing and processing stories and explored a variety of ways of using them. This was not a simple linear process of deciding what was needed and selecting the methods to get there. The MI work was influenced by the development of ideas and perceptions of what was possible, who was involved, timing and serendipity (e.g. engaged patients and key staff with particular skills and time to allocate to the project).

The challenge of capturing an authentic user experience to form the starting point of an information project was often a practical one. There needed to be time and space for users to become comfortable with one another and with staff, and to exchange stories (as one user put it, what was needed was *a nice space and a bit of lunch*). The structure of the user event had to be such that both positive and negative experiences were captured and reflected on. In addition, there had to be an atmosphere of genuine interest in, and valuing of, the user experience.

Not everyone is a natural performer in front of the camera, especially if their condition affects their appearance, their speech, their cognitive abilities or their emotions. Some users with stroke needed one-to-one support from a speech and language therapist to be confident to take part. Multimedia tools allowed flexibility in how messages were conveyed. For example, the use of subtitles allowed those with indistinct speech to communicate clearly, and in other cases, the person was only filmed from behind to protect their identity. It was made clear to all users that they could withdraw at any point and that if they changed their mind their contribution would be erased.

It is worth commenting that stories are inherently emotionally charged, especially when they concern illness and healthcare.[7] At times, meetings whose purpose was to capture stories quickly began to focus on the emotional response to having a stroke. Meetings sometimes swung from silence to anger to humour – and required skilled facilitation both to manage the emotional currents and deliver on the task of making the film.

Some people could be quite challenging and forthright, but I thought that was quite good because they were open about the frustrations they'd experienced and their needs as well. (Project worker, SIAG)

Challenge 3: Deciding on content and style

Whilst clinicians and patients may agree on some (and even most) of the content of an information leaflet or DVD, our experience suggests that there will be many arguments about the detail and how it is presented. In general, clinicians tended to want to include a lot of factual detail and felt strongly about clinical accuracy. Users, on the other hand, wanted simple, direct messages and the opportunity to access more information if necessary.

> *It was quite difficult to keep a balance because when I took the script to clinicians it didn't sound clinical enough for them. When I took it to the patients, it was too clinical. The clinicians were watching the DVD for clinical accuracy, such as how a patient was dialysing, they couldn't see the bigger picture.* (Information Officer, kidney MI)

In relation to this issue, there is an interesting paper about producing course materials for an Open University module on mental health.[8] The authors describe a struggle between clinicians who wanted to 'balance' service users' accounts with their own more clinically oriented commentary, whereas the users wanted their experiences to stand alone as an anthology without professional viewpoints, which they feared would devalue the user contributions and dilute their impact. The decision was a difficult one but the course developers agreed to let the users' accounts stand.

A common perception amongst clinicians was that *'we give information, we tell people again and again'*, but the service users often said things like *'I didn't know, no-one told me that'*. To some extent, both these perceptions are true, and they highlight that unless the right amount of the right type of information is offered at the right point in the illness journey, there will be a mismatch between what the patient *should* know and what they actually *do* know.

There is, of course, no 'ideal' amount of content or best method of presenting it, since people have different information needs and learning styles. But in our experience, patients wanted things presented in short, simple terms with jargon removed. Clinicians are often so steeped in jargon that they do not notice it, and are often surprised when lay people have difficulty understanding what for them are familiar terms.

> *Undoubtedly having service users involved in those negotiations has been very powerful . . . diverse groups of people . . . Some people are very confident to challenge, particularly once they've got a sense that they're*

going to be listened to and respected ... sometimes it's less overt. But getting patients and clinicians to work together ... the way patients talk about or perceive something that's been developed indicates very clearly how it will come over to the patients who will be using it. (Service improvement lead, kidney MI)

The sexual health project consulted service users and clinicians separately. Clinicians had strong views on what content should be included, and the leaflets went through some expensive reprints because the tensions between perspectives were not resolved at the pre-design stage. Reflecting on this after the end of the project, the project team commented that focus groups of staff and users had proved unworkable for various reasons, but wondered whether they might have invited clinicians to test out the draft leaflets with patients in their own clinics to get across the message that the information, whilst accurate, was not meaningful or engaging to users.

Clinicians working on information projects often spoke about the problem of 'denial' – patients not wanting (or not being ready for) potentially upsetting information.

So there's that battle between what patients want to know and what we feel they need to know, whether they want to know it or not. And that was almost impossible to compromise on. At times we did just make the decision not to listen to what patients had said, maybe that negates the whole point of user involvement. (Nurse, kidney MI)

As the above example shows, information that is considered potentially upsetting must be treated particularly carefully, and clinicians and users sometimes disagreed on how and when such information should be presented. A good example of this was when kidney patients felt that 'supportive care' (i.e. no active treatment) should be included as an option in the DVD about 'dialysis choices'. Clinicians were initially reluctant, since from the perspective of most doctors and nurses, end stage kidney disease is a treatable condition. The patients, however, felt that being on dialysis (and/or a transplant list) is physically and emotionally draining, and that a very reasonable choice for *some* people would be to allow the kidney disease to run its natural course with what amounted to palliative care. Doctors countered that the target audience for the DVD was people in *early* kidney disease, and a 'no treatment' option would frighten many people unnecessarily. After much heated discussion it was agreed that the section on 'no treatment' would be made available on the DVD but prefaced with advice to viewers that they should only continue to watch if they were considering this option. Staff training also emphasised selective viewing of the DVD.

Decisions on style and format were difficult to make, and assistance from professional (or semi-professional designers) was sometimes invaluable. We found that starting with an example, rather than an abstract idea, often allowed discussants to move on to an acceptable design.

> *I remember J– at one of the meetings showing a mock up of what a picture card might look like, and examples from elsewhere. And certainly the group was positive with that. So it was starting off with something for people to comment on and give their feedback on and whether they thought it would be useful.* (Information officer, kidney MI)

We found that the design process was an iterative one, and required regular input from users and staff. A model which worked well in the stroke project was a small, committed panel who would provide rapid feedback on draft materials, combined with wider testing of materials at a later stage in the process. One staff member was responsible for maintaining interest and commitment from the core panel, for example by ensuring that people were kept informed:

> *The importance of getting back to people. You've had a meeting and do some minutes straightaway and tell them what's happening. If you've produced something, let them have a copy of what's been produced. I think we've learnt just how important that was, particularly to keep people engaged and believing in you. A few people said, which was quite nice, 'Oh I've been involved in things before and it was all talking and nothing happened'. So when you went back to them for something else, they were happy to contribute.* (Project worker, stroke MI)

We found that debate and disagreement on the emerging designs was generally a positive and creative force:

> *Debate was important. Sometimes I knew what I wanted but things would go off on a bit of a tangent, but that was actually okay, because sometimes just listening – they would be talking and me jotting down notes and thinking – so they weren't giving me bullet points of what*

they wanted. Sometimes their experiences and just talking through what happened to them gave me the clues about what they needed. But it wouldn't have worked with just service users. We had health-care professionals there some of the time. I took information to them as well and we were developing information, because it needed to work for them and to fit in with what they were doing, and to ensure that it was accurate. So that was a real support.' (Project worker, stroke MI)

In relation to wider consultation, the kidney MI made use of a ready 'panel' in the dialysis units where they offered chapters of a booklet to all patients attending for dialysis. These people often had very different levels of interest and health literacy from the self-selected group who had contributed actively to the core panel.

I think the greatest contribution was when patients were reviewing the DVD and the book. Reading it, watching it, giving feedback about how it made them feel . . . that led to changes and it was very useful. (Nurse, kidney MI)

This and other examples of feedback from 'unselected' samples of users highlight the wide range of health literacy amongst service users in all the projects. In relation to DVD development, the visual dimensions of health literacy may be overlooked because the focus in research is usually on people's ability to comprehend written materials. But Entwhistle et al. have shown that carefully selected visual and spoken material, including images, diagrams and so on may help enhance understanding in those less able to deal with written materials.[9]

Challenge 4: Timing and budget

The previous section hopefully conveys that co-designing and co-producing information is often a slow and non-linear process. We found that many of the initiatives that were subsequently hailed as highly successful went far beyond their original timescale and budget because we had not anticipated the level of input needed to get the designs right and refine them optimally.

The various kidney DVD projects found that individual patient in-terviews were very time-consuming but were the best way of get-ting patients to talk about themselves and their views on dialysis, yielding a breadth and richness of information that underpinned the DVD. They had initially been advised to run focus groups *'to find out what patients know'*, but the project worker soon realised that this method would not have provided the rich, personal narratives that made the final product so authentic and accessible.

The desire to produce the best design and test it on as wide a spectrum of users as possible must, of course, be balanced against real deadlines and budgets. The MI teams were fortunate in having generous (though not unlimited) funding, but we recognise that many teams developing information products with users do not have this luxury. However, as this experience shows, involving users throughout the process will ensure than any information produced will deliver value for money.

The time input of patients must also be taken into account, especially if their illness is potentially compromising. In the stroke project, for example, there was quite a turnover because of health problems. A few found it difficult to cope with being in meetings. The information group learnt early on not to 'overwork' these individuals (and hence, not invite them to too many meetings!). They found that for the information projects, people with cognitive impairments could work at home with the help of a carer and make a valuable input.

Challenge 5: Seeing how the information is used

The initial focus of all the information projects in the MI was on producing materials. But once produced, an equally important dimension was whether and how the materials were actually used. The stroke information team, for example, followed up the use of a handbook they produced for stroke patients and gave out on the wards. Research appeared to indicate that some people thought the handbook was just for while they were in hospital, and some appeared to treat it as a picture book to browse through rather than as a hands-on practical handbook. Some felt it was too good to take home with them *'you couldn't possibly be giving this to me'*.

This finding highlighted the need for the stroke information group to do more educational work with staff to introduce them to the handbook and get them to encourage patients to use it actively both on the ward and when they went home, and also for staff to recognise that carers had different information needs (and sometimes, different learning styles) to patients. Subsequently, patient surveys from hospital wards were more positive, with many people saying they had been given the handbook. Input at senior management level helped – the handbook is now embedded in the patient survey which is routinely carried out on the stroke unit. Patients are asked 'did you receive the handbook and was it explained to you?' It is also included in the handover between shifts via a tick box question 'has the patient been given a copy?'.

Summary: Ten tips for effective co-production of information

1 Make the user experience the starting point of co-produced materials. This is where your users are the experts.

2 Users' personal stories are likely to be engaging and powerful but often need careful editing – a task which requires skill and sensitivity.

3 The development pathway for any co-produced materials is likely to be long and non-linear. Try to build in time and budget to reflect this.

4 Recruit a core group of users and clinicians to serve as an advisory panel, and identify a wider audience representing a range of learning styles and literacy levels for testing later drafts.

5 Get staff and users together to hammer out their disagreements on content and style before the materials are published, otherwise expensive reprints may be needed. Anticipate that clinicians will focus on clinical facts whereas users will want short, clear messages and an explanation of things that matter to them.

6 When covering sensitive issues (such as life-threatening complications) or significant healthcare choices (such as what sort of dialysis to opt for), anticipate that users and clinicians may disagree strongly on both content and style.

7 Seek input from people with professional design skills if possible. Good visuals and diagrams can sometimes overcome limitations in health literacy and help to achieve accommodation between conflicting perspectives.

8 Follow through after publication to see how (if at all) the materials are being used and take steps to maximise distribution and support for using the materials actively.

9 Recognise that input to information projects can be physically and emotionally demanding for patients, and provide appropriate flexibility and support.

10 Ensure that clinical, managerial and administration staff (as appropriate) are trained to be aware of and understand user-generated materials so that they can promote their use.

References

1. Coulter A, Ellins J, Swain D, Clarke A, Heron P, Rasul F et al. *Assessing the Quality of Information to Support People in Making Decisions About Their Health and Healthcare.* Oxford: Picker Institute; 2006.

2. Edgman-Levitan S, Cleary PD. What information do consumers want and need? *Health Aff* 1996; 15(4):42–56.

3. Jennings BM, Heiner SL, Loan LA, Hemman EA, Swanson KM. What really matters to healthcare consumers. *J Nurs Adm* 2005; 35(4):173–180.

4. Swain D, Ellins J, Coulter A, Heron P, Howell E, McGee H et al. *Accessing Information About Health and Social Care Services.* Oxford: Picker Institute; 2007.

5. Coulter A, Parsons S, Askham J. *Where Are the Patients in Decision-Making About Their Own Care?* Geneva: World Health Organisation; 2008.

6. Marshall M, Noble J, Davies H, Waterman H, Walshe K, Sheaff R et al. Development of an information source for patients and the public about general practice services: an action research study. *Health Exp* 2006; 9: 265–274.

7. Greenhalgh T, Hurwitz B. Narrative based medicine: why study narrative? *BMJ* 1999; 318(7175):48–50.

8. Reynolds J, Read J. Opening minds: user involvement in the production of learning materials on mental health and distress. *Soc Work Educ* 1999; 18(4):417–431.

9. Entwhistle V, Williams B. Health literacy: the need to consider images as well as words. *Health Exp* 2008; 11:99–101.

CHAPTER 6

Involving users in leadership and governance

Fran Woodard[1], Lizzy Bovill[2] & David Freedman[3]
[1]Integrated Cancer Centre, King's Health Partners, London, UK
[2]London Ambulance Service NHS Trust, London, UK
[3]Freelance writer, London, UK

Leadership is a term that eludes definition.[1,2] Concepts of leadership include the charismatic leader (e.g. Martin Luther King or Barack Obama) who through impassioned rhetoric aim to inspire change.[3] By contrast, the focus of 'transformational leadership' (the model chosen by the modernisation initiative (MI)) is not on a particular leader but on empowering all staff to grasp leadership and engender change in organisations at all levels.[4]

Transformational leadership is about setting long-term goals and strong values, and encouraging a culture of empowerment for everyone involved at all levels. It can potentially effect both large changes (in strategy and approach) and small changes (in particular practices) in an organisation, oriented to improving outcomes for users. For example, if a nurse finds a way to reduce the waiting times in an outpatient clinic and shares this improvement with colleagues and supports its implementation, this demonstrates transformational leadership. Or if a group of service users describe a radical new vision for their ideal service and work with staff to deliver this, all involved could be described as 'transformational leaders'.

There has been no shortage of leadership initiatives in the National Health Service (NHS) over the past 10 years. The NHS Plan, published in 2000,[5] mandated the creation of the Leadership

User Involvement in Health Care, 1st edition. Edited by Trisha Greenhalgh, Charlotte Humphrey and Fran Woodard. © 2011 Blackwell Publishing Ltd.

Agency, which soon merged into the NHS Modernisation Agency, which in turn morphed into the NHS Institute of Innovation and Improvement. In 2008, Health Minister Lord Darzi wrote eloquently on the need to develop leadership capacity in the NHS in the white paper *High Quality Care For All*.[6] Partly as a response to this, the NHS Leadership Council was introduced in April 2009 with a brief to promote the transformation of leadership capability and capacity. A recent independent report highlighted the need to ensure this Council manages a number of 'complex dualities' including the need to empower frontline staff to become transformational leaders, create co-ordinated values and principles at all levels and inspire change in the system where it has failed before.[7] These periodic reorganisations beg the question of what is it that prevents leadership flourishing, and what behaviours and cultures inhibit the development of transformational leadership.[8]

Transformational leadership allowed the MI to go beyond usual lay membership (e.g. non-executive directors of NHS trusts) to include and develop users as leaders in a range of different ways and at many different levels, creating opportunities for them to move from being 'consumers' to 'creators' of services. As the examples below illustrate, service users sometimes took on leadership roles at the most senior levels and made long-term commitments; others held more limited roles in smaller projects, but still had significant impact on the culture and behaviour of the projects.

Closely related to leadership is the role of service users in governance – that is, in helping ensure the accountability of the programme and determining whether projects are fulfilling their remits (see Chapter 2 for details of the governance structures). Through being directly involved in governance and leadership roles, users were able to help shape the projects by bringing perspectives that went far beyond those understood by clinicians and managers; they challenged service provision, helped design improvements and were a part of the assessment process to evaluate improvement initiatives. The service user brings insights from actually using the service; he or she is able to plot the experience of the journey through each service contact and to experience these as continuous rather than discrete and detached events.[9] Coping with managing a disease (such as kidney disease) or with the consequences of an acute event (such as a stroke) may well be a permanent part of a person's life. Consequently, users become experts on many different aspects of illness and its treatment.[10]

Traditionally, this has rarely been understood or appreciated by service providers.

> *Like most patients, despite being a potentially invaluable resource, I have rarely felt equal in the consultation room; rarely been able to share my experiences to help others; rarely offered a chance to feedback as a 'consumer' of services. As a patient, for nearly a quarter of century, I had no real voice.* (Service user, kidney MI)

The MI's ambitious goal was to change this culture and build a genuine partnership so that users could influence fundamentally the way professionals thought about the services in which they worked. The MI Board (which did not have user representation itself – see Challenge 1 below) held the individual programme managers and their Steering Groups accountable for ensuring user involvement and engagement at all levels, including on their boards and working groups. Below, we offer two contrasting examples – one from the kidney MI and one from the stroke MI – before discussing some challenges that cut across all the projects. As set out in Chapter 3, the sexual health MI faced particular challenges in relation to user involvement since being a 'user of sexual health services' did not engender the same kind of long-term commitment and identification that being a user of stroke or kidney services did. For these reasons, service users were not directly involved in the management and governance of that project. However, both the mystery shopper initiative (see Chapter 3) and the presence of third-sector groups (e.g. Brook Advisory Service, Terrence Higgins Trust and various local advocacy groups for sexual minorities) on the sexual Health Project Management Board provided indirect user input to the governance of the programme.

Example 1: A patient chair in the Kidney MI Steering Group

Chronic kidney disease is a lifelong condition. Relationships between patients and staff are often intense and can last for decades, though they may change substantially over time depending on the treatment regimen. They are sometimes characterised by a high degree of dependence, which may make users reluctant to criticise services. Power relationships are complex and unequal, although many patients and carers develop a high level of specialised medical and technical expertise.

Services for people with kidney disease were offered at a number of locations across South East London and Kent and were co-ordinated by two foundation NHS Foundation Trusts. Staff from the two hospitals were brought together on the Kidney MI Steering Group which planned and oversaw service improvements and redesign. It was decided at the outset to invite users who represented a wide range of illness experience and treatment modalities. A patient, J, who had lived with kidney disease for most of his life was recommended by the kidney consultant and invited to chair the Steering Group, which had about 20 members. The management structure was described as 'triumvirate' (i.e. patient chair, clinical lead and programme manager) The group included several other users but we focus here on the role and influence of the chair (Figure 6.1).

J was eager to be involved and fulfilled the key criteria of 'user expertise':[10] he had long personal experience of the disease, had been through a large range of treatments, had a deep understanding of his disease clinically and practically, and now played a very active role in his treatment. He was also highly intelligent, educated and articulate, and insisted on being treated as a partner in his treatment. His consultant saw him as someone who took responsibility for his illness and was not afraid to challenge and discuss his

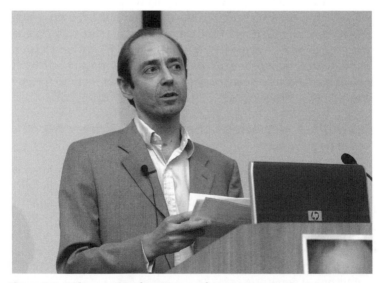

Figure 6.1 Kidney patient lecturing on the user experience.

treatment options. Being both willing and able to challenge clinical staff, J had great potential to challenge the established culture and power base within kidney services.

The consultant who recommended J was also responsible for his clinical care; he was also the Director of Kidney Services for one of the trusts and a member of the Kidney MI Steering Group. These multiple roles complicated the 'doctor–patient' relationship since J's role in the leadership and governance of the project placed him in a position of power *over* his own clinician – yet at the same time the nature of his illness created a degree of personal vulnerability. It is to the consultant's credit that he deliberately recommended a patient with a history of challenging the status quo.

> *What was key [to the success of my role] was that from the start, the lead clinicians and the MI staff at all levels showed a strong commitment to the role itself, and myself as Chair, recognising that working with patients as peers required time and effort – for it was a new experience for all of us!* (J, Chair of Kidney MI Steering Group)

The role of the Chair of the Steering Group (Box 6.1) was not just to conduct the business of the meetings and ensure that the agenda items were covered, but also to keep the longer term aims, objectives and governance of the project in mind and hold other members of the Group to account for delivering on them. A Chair who is also a patient must be able to maintain balance and neutrality, contributing a crucial patient perspective while also going beyond the role of patients' advocate when needed. Even the mundane business of keeping the Group in order was challenging at first for a layperson who was perceived by some members first as a patient and only secondly as a chair. This became less of an issue as J became more experienced in the role.

Every organisation has its own cultures and subcultures, so part of the task of learning to be a chairperson is learning the appropriate modes of behaviour and forms of interaction in order to be accepted and effective. By positioning a patient in the Chair, 'normal' culture in this kidney service was disrupted and innovative ways of operating were required from the outset.

> *I think the patients can give words to people's feelings for their peers much better than anyone else can … J can put into words things other people can't and I think he's much better at doing that than us.* (Senior clinician, Kidney MI)

Box 6.1 Role description for Chair of the Kidney MI Steering Group

- Lead and Chair discussions relevant to the development of the programme at the Steering Group with the support of the Programme Manager.
- Ensure the programme remains focused on the achievement of the vision
- Ensure the work is benefiting all patients from Lambeth and Southwark no matter where their care is based (home, hospital, General practitioner (GP), satellite unit).
- Help encourage the involvement of patients and carers at every level of the programme.
- Ensure the work remains innovative and radical, resulting in changes that benefit patients, staff and the community
- Lead strategic discussions on the development of the workstreams, and the interaction and integration between workstreams and with other modernisation initiative programmes.
- Provide leadership in ensuring transparency of the programme, evaluation of workstreams and generating learning at each stage
- Ensure the programme meets work plan targets and deadlines and is accountable for expenditure
- Help manage and resolve problems or conflict within or between organisations, individuals or groups
- Be one of a number of public faces of the programme, including speaking at conferences or in communication or marketing publications
- Be adaptable in light of the needs of the programme in agreement with the Programme Manager.

In setting up any new processes, relationships or ways of working there are inevitably tensions. J forced new ideas and approaches, which challenged ways of thinking but also disrupted normal governance or meeting processes. Despite his need to acquire new skills (in chairing) and knowledge (of the structure and organisation of the NHS and local services), J nevertheless had significant power both by virtue of being a service user and by being positioned *outside* the normal NHS governance framework – hence he was able to question taken for granted assumptions and challenge conventional approaches to governance and leadership.

> *I had absolutely no idea how the NHS worked, how decisions were made, how the NHS decided which services to fund. I had barely a passing knowledge of basic NHS concepts, such as 'Patient Pathway', the seemingly very confusing distinction between 'primary' and 'secondary' care – or indeed, the vital, but seemingly invisible role of commissioners.*(J, kidney patient and Chair of Kidney MI Steering Group)

All members of the Steering Group had a sense of anxiety at the outset. J was anxious that he did not possess the appropriate knowledge and skills to be an effective chair; the managers were concerned that the relatively tough way that they sometimes behaved towards each other might not be considered appropriate with patients and carers present and the clinicians were concerned about raising clinical issues in front of patients. Also, clinicians' experience of patients expressing their views was largely limited to complaints, and patients were largely ignorant of the complex infrastructure and organisation that underpins the front-line service.

One consequence of this was that both J and the Programme Manager had to spend *'phenomenal amounts of time'* (MI Director) to ensure that J was sufficiently well briefed on (for example) the way NHS services were structured, how the two Primary Care Trusts, two specialist secondary and tertiary referral Foundation Trusts operated and interfaced, the vocabulary of the NHS, and how the processes (planning, commissioning and running) of the relevant aspects of the NHS functioned. No one knew beforehand how much time this would take. We found that in the first year, training J took 1 day per month (5% of a working week) plus a half day premeeting before each board meeting, plus the time that J was giving to other segments of the kidney programme of the MI. This was a substantial commitment, both for the Programme Manager and for J, especially as it took him away from his professional, income-generating work.

> *In terms of Chair, I don't think I realised how much of my time it would take to educate and develop J in a chairing role . . . . . . he had no previous experience of management of the NHS therefore didn't understand the*

management structure of organisations, how decisions are made within any of the NHS organisations, what the interactions are like between different clinicians. His experiences of business and the health service have been very top down, very medical directed. And I think he thought that was how decisions were made and so he very quickly realised that actually it's a lot about influence and it's a lot about negotiation and it's not directive in that way.(Programme manager)

There were palpable tensions between the members of the triumvirate management structure at times. For example, J wanted the initiative to focus on developing a more holistic approach to improving quality of life for kidney patients, including offering complementary therapies. Clinicians were sceptical of complementary approaches. All parties were encouraged to argue their perspective and a range of evidence was discussed. In the end, a short pilot for reflexology with dialysis patients was undertaken.

Over time, the Steering Group developed a new code of conduct that was different from other NHS committees and from the ways of working that the service user members had previously experienced. The service users gained a greater understanding of how the NHS worked, how treatments are structured, how to function effectively on a NHS committee, and were able to give unique input into the various projects. The NHS members of the Steering Group, both managers and clinicians, gained a far greater understanding of patients and their lives, of which their disease and its treatment forms only a part. Thus, for example, the clinicians learned about the emotional impact that polycystic kidney disease (an inherited condition) can have on a large family where different family members are at different stages of the disease (healthy, on dialysis, living with a transplant or having had a failed transplant).[9]

As the programme evolved, all members of the Steering Group gained in confidence and mutual trust and respect. This did not mean that disagreements and tensions evaporated (far from it), but it did mean that issues could be talked through in a more open and constructive way, with mutual respect, and were more likely to be resolved creatively in ways that led to better results.

> ... *the clinicians were very nervous about actually highlighting difficulties or problems in that meeting with patients there, whether they were chairing or just members......but as the clinicians, managers and patients have got more used to working together, they're much*

*better at challenging each other now and more willing to have more
open conversations in that context because…..they trust each other
more. Having a patient in the chair has really helped us focus on the
SU experience and overcome cultural barriers that have prevented us
from improving it.*(Kidney MI Steering Group member)

*I think it's been about developing a cultural change in the staff, that
they feel more accountable to the patients, and I think that the patients
feel empowered to challenge, and the staff are more open to challenge
than perhaps they were before the programme.* (Programme manager, Kidney MI)

Whilst J remained committed to the Steering Group throughout the
MI, there was a turnover of other service users, who left for various
reasons including outside pressures, change in treatment (e.g.
kidney transplant operation) and general health. The need for an
ongoing recruitment process of service users and induction for new
members took up a substantial amount of the Programme Manager's time.

*It's a continuous struggle to make sure that you have a range of patients
on the steering group. And that you continue to have a range of patients
with a range of experiences. And that sometimes it's been a challenge
to try and make sure that we had the range and not just all from one
group.* (Programme manager)

Given the turnover of other users, the continuity in user perspective
provided by the Chair was particularly valuable, and sent an
important message to those outside of the initiative. The 'novelty'
of a patient chair attracted attention to the work both locally and
nationally. It also meant that other service user members felt confident
from the outset that they could contribute to projects in a
way that went beyond tokenism. As a result the programme gained
credibility with commissioners, providers, staff, clinicians and other
service users. At times, this provided crucial leverage with decision
makers:

In a conference speech towards the end of the MI, J summed up
what he felt were the advantages and disadvantages for clinicians
of employing a patient chair:

*The advantages include ensuring you articulate a clear vision of change
that gets both patient and clinician buy-in; helping ensure the proposed
changes always focus on improving the actual quality of life of*

the patient; ensuring all the patient and staff voices are heard; an independent voice that can unite individuals together and diffuse organisational conflict; a critical friend that can help ensure changes are not just superficial, but if needed, radical; and a symbol to other patients, staff and stakeholders, that high level service user engagement is a reality.

The disadvantages include a need [for you clinicians] to 'ring fence' valuable time to bridge the initial patient-clinician skill gap; to genuinely partner with someone you might normally consider an 'outsider'; to share decision making with someone who might not always, quite, see things your way; and to be accountable to a service user chair for your projects' finances and outcomes. (J, kidney patient and Chair, Kidney MI Steering Group)

In a separate interview, J highlighted the learning and personal growth he gained from his involvement.

For me personally it has been challenging, hard work but inspirational. No – not just inspirational: life changing. (J, kidney patient and Chair, Kidney MI Steering Group)

After the end of the MI, J went on to become an active member of the Steering Group in an end-of-life care project, the Patient and Carer Steering Group and the NHS Alliance Patient and Public Involvement Steering Group.

Example 2: Leadership and governance in the stroke pathway

Stroke care involves prevention, acute care (usually in hospital) and rehabilitation (usually in the community). A number of different NHS trusts, other statutory agencies and the voluntary and private sectors all provide services for people who have suffered a stroke. A major challenge for stroke services in the MI was achieving coordination between all these providers and stakeholders to ensure consistency of standards around a single, common care pathway and avoid fragmentation or duplication. Input of service users was actively sought in focus groups and consultation events (see Chapter 3), and in principle user involvement in leadership and governance was supported, but because of the complexity of the service model, it was not felt appropriate to involve users in such roles until the programme had established its core structure and agreed on what the common approach would look like.

Different people in the stroke MI had differing perspectives on what 'engagement' and 'leadership' from service users would mean and where it would add value. Some thought users could be involved in all aspects of the programme; others that users had very little to add. Reflecting after the end of the MI, some senior staff who had been opposed to early user involvement felt in retrospect that this might have helped accelerate the development of strong service user leadership capability within the professional group. At the time however, it would have meant that service users would have had to spend a lot of time on the programme's basic structure and resolving local political differences, rather than have direct input to the design or evaluation of services.

A year after the programme began, the core team felt it was sufficiently clear in its direction to be ready to bring users on board in governance structures and leadership roles. The bar had already been set at a high level by the Kidney MI (see previous example), so tokenistic representation was not seen as appropriate. The Stroke MI aspired to authentic engagement, but this posed substantial challenges in a less mature programme where there were significant complexities (cross-organisational cultures, secondary versus primary care priorities, health versus social care objectives, service user aspirations of recovery etc.) and different ideas of how to achieve the vision.

As described in Chapter 3, informal join-in sessions were set up to which service users of all ages were invited to attend. They were invited to join in a variety of ways: strategic, leadership, governance, and to *tell us your story and what we can do to make a difference* (Senior Manager, Stroke MI). These events took place in a neutral space belonging to the voluntary sector and the events were made 'aphasia friendly' (aphasia is the loss of previously acquired skills of speaking and writing, understanding and reading, which occurs fairly commonly in stroke), transport was laid on and food was provided in order to help create a welcoming atmosphere.

As in the Kidney MI example above, efforts were made to attract people from different ages, backgrounds and illness experience, and different volunteers took on roles at different levels and for different periods of time. We found that agreement and clarity was essential on what was expected from the service user and from the staff with

Box 6.2 Checklist for induction to Stroke MI Steering Group

- What is the Stroke MI aiming to do?
- How long will it last?
- Where is it happening?
- Who is doing it?
- What the project is not doing
- How is the project organised – leadership, governance, structures of work areas, staff
- Who is on the Steering Group and what is their role?
- What does the Steering Group do?
- How does the Steering Group work?
- What will the role of a service user be on the Steering Group?
- Confirm enthusiasm and desire to contribute (more important than previous experience)
- How to access training?

whom they would be working. Box 6.2 shows a checklist for the induction process.

These early efforts to involve, train and coordinate service user input to leadership and governance were time-consuming and initially appeared to bear little fruit.[11] Only three users initially came forward who were interested in being involved in the Steering Group and one soon withdrew because of carer commitments. A second wave of recruitment yielded one further user who, after two or three sessions, stopped attending with no reason given. One person felt unable to join the Steering Group as one side effect of his stroke was that he tended to cry at times and found this very difficult to manage in public situations; staff were unable to reassure him sufficiently that this could be accommodated.

The original two users remained with the Steering Group for the duration of the MI and both took on additional roles leading individual workstreams (one, for example, led 'Living with a Disability' where he championed user involvement by others living with stroke). Both were men, highly skilled and successful in their careers. One, H, was an industrialist, and businessman and carer; the other, N, had a background in the public sector and considerable experience in qualitative assessment and facilitation. Both were offered payment for their input and one accepted a daily consultancy rate for his role in leading an individual workstream; the other refused such payment on the grounds that he '*just wanted to make a difference*'. The issue of payment is taken up in Chapter 7.

Training for these members included both factual knowledge about how services worked and also confidence-building and assuring users that their contribution mattered and was valued. Meeting papers were adapted to ensure they were user friendly (with a minimum of jargon or acronyms), in each user's preferred medium (e.g. large font). In addition, as in the Kidney MI, the service users had a detailed meeting with the Programme Manager before each Steering Group meeting so that they could receive clarification on any issues and consider what they thought about the various agenda items. The users were made aware of the different perspectives on an item or decision to be made, the pros and cons, and the potential ramifications. Having time to understand complex issues in advance of the meetings allowed the users to air ideas, question and challenge, and formulate a view (or not) without the intense pressure of being in the meeting.

In addition, senior staff ensured that users' anxieties (e.g. concerns about being put on the spot, communication difficulties, not understanding the whole context or individual projects or issues, not always having to have a view or comment to make, appearing to criticise clinicians or healthcare staff, not being listened to, not adding value) were appreciated by other group members who modified their behaviour in the meetings accordingly. These preparatory measures (both cognitive and emotional) were particularly important for involving stroke service users who may have communication or cognitive deficits and, consequently, may feel especially vulnerable, and their confidence grew significantly with time.

Training sessions for other Steering Group members on how to co-create strategy and governance with service users were also planned. However, because of logistical difficulties this was ultimately squeezed into a short slot on one of the management group agendas, and therefore was not as useful as it might have been.

Users, like other group members, come with a range of individual skills and experiences which influence the contribution that they make to leadership. The skills the two service users brought to the Steering Group were very different. H had a background in finance and felt most confident helping to bring clarity to concrete areas such as budgets, costings, spending projections, etc. H was also an active member of a local stroke support group and played a pivotal role in engaging this group in the programme of work, and briefing them on the programme's aims, approaches and achievements. N, on the other hand, came from a public sector background and was more comfortable in the culture of the programme and helping to facilitate the processes of the Steering Group.

For both of them, sitting on a formal decision-making board that included clinicians and contributing to discussions of health strategy was a new experience.

> *It was a unique experience. I mean, I've never been in a room with lots of clinicians, going into an environment where you didn't under-stand the context or the language, you really have to learn it fairly quickly. . . . . .I used to pick them up and say, 'I don't know what that means?' which was in itself challenging. . . .and get them to talk to me about the jargon they were actually using. . . .But, it was daunting and I think I was very uncomfortable initially. . . .I've got good communica-tion skills, so I was potentially a good option in a way as someone who could go on there, and was fairly familiar with what was going on. I suppose over a period of time, I've actually learnt a great deal about stroke and the way stroke services are provided and who's involved, and that whole area of the stroke.* (N, patient with a public sector background and member of Stroke MI Steering Group)

The service users were there to bring their personal experiences and expertise, but they were not elected representatives, nor were they selected as in some way 'representative' of stroke service users in general. One of the users acknowledged this issue:

> *I just made what I thought were going to be useful points for stroke patients generally and I don't think I necessarily saw myself as repre-senting them, I just wanted to ensure that whenever I did say anything, it. . . .could benefit other stroke users as well. . . . the important thing is that people are given a voice and the opportunity to say what they want to say regardless of what the condition is. . . .that they're given their space and time to actually voice an opinion and record it and, you know, hopefully be listened to and possibly being acted on as well.* (N, patient with a public sector background and member of Stroke MI Steering Group)

N is describing what Martin called 'ordinary people bringing or-dinary knowledge',[10] with great authenticity given his personal experience of the condition. Users' personal narratives also contributed a great deal of understanding about the clinical aspects of their condition and the complexity of the structure and organisation of services from the user's perspective. As some professional Steering Group members put it:

> *Having users on the Steering Group was a positive and yet challenging experience. There were specific needs around language, their level of understanding and making sure their voice is heard.*
>
> *I just think ...... how valuable the service user's background (was)...... H was great on finances, he's been very interesting and very pragmatic around the reality of life [following a stroke]. N has a huge [public sector] background and I think we forget that they add in huge benefits (because of their backgrounds and their) different perspectives.* (Professional members, Stroke MI Steering Group)

Within the stroke MI, historical context and local politics within and across stroke services played a significant part. Because of this, the MI Director chaired the Stroke MI Steering Group. She held a senior management position and was seen as relatively non-aligned in a highly complex and political environment. These meetings were challenging, with many valid but conflicting priorities and perspectives. Chairing complex multi-stakeholder meetings with users as members presented professional and personal challenges for the MI Director; her reflections and learning from this experience are summarised in Box 6.3. A key issue was how to balance giving space to the user voice and empowering users to contribute, whilst also ensuring efficient and effective formal processes, keeping to time and being realistic and pragmatic about budget and priorities. Users sometimes felt that the programme was not stretching far enough, or needed significant changes. But there was not always the capacity, capability, resources, or sphere of influence to deliver on these suggestions.

A noticeable feature of the Stroke MI Steering Group was how it changed over time. Members' behaviour at the meetings began to reflect greater acceptance and consideration for the users; the pace of the meetings slowed down, allowing not just users but others within the group to be heard and a range of opinions aired; and power bases also began to shift. As the programme became more mature, many 'routine' issues came to be dealt with outside the Steering Group, leaving more time for contentious, complex and ambiguous issues to be addressed. Also with time, the users gained in confidence and felt increasingly able to challenge the professionals in quite direct ways.

Box 6.3 Reflections from the MI Director of chairing a complex multi-stakeholder steering group including service users:

- Preparation for the pre-brief with users is key. Need to consider the agenda and likely direction of discussion. The pre-briefing facilitates an understanding of the users' perspective and flags issues they are likely to raise, as well as explaining other perspectives to the users, which helps to enable a constructive debate within the Steering Group. Meeting de-briefs may also be beneficial
- Ensure that all members get time to speak and are facilitated to be able to contribute
- Listen differently. Users bring completely new mindsets and perspectives (e.g. on quality of life), and their agenda may seem irrelevant until the group have 'unlearnt' the rules for what is relevant. Enabling and facilitating this is a key role of the Chair.
- Ensure clarity and understanding about the governance procedures which need to be adhered to. This can help direction with very complex agendas
- Systematic strategies are needed when members (including but not limited to service users) stray from the agenda or focus of the discussion or are very verbose. The same strategy should be applied for all members, taking into consideration any communication difficulties
- Prepare carefully and brief all members for complex, difficult or contentious agenda items
- Ensure that service users are constructively challenged in broadly the same way as professional members are (as long as they have been fully prepared and briefed). At times this is difficult and uncomfortable, but can be done constructively and is key for the governance of the Steering Group
- Challenge inappropriate behaviour (e.g. single-issue campaigning) either within the group or by following up outside the meeting.
- Have confidence in the process: service user involvement gets much easier with time.

As with the Kidney MI, the presence of service users on the Stroke Steering Group gave the programme credibility with other users in the area, which meant that it received more feedback from other users. This wider feedback was fed back into the work programme in different ways.

Perhaps because of their long-term involvement with the Stroke MI and the skills, experience and confidence they accumulated, the service users achieved significant gains in some strategic areas. N, for example, attended critical meetings to address the sustainability of projects in partner organisations and supported proposals for mainstreaming of services that had been initiated by the MI. This was a compelling message to be heard from a service user, especially within a debate focussed on affordability and financial models of care. N ensured the patient experience was retained at the core of a vital business proposal. Reflecting on his experiences at the end of the project, he expressed a sense of fulfilment and personal gain:

> ... it's been really good. I've really enjoyed it and I've met some great people who I will continue to have contact with beyond the MI. And it's been very positive. What I've found particularly meaningful for me has been my work .... The idea of actually going out and meeting other people who have had strokes. ..... what's possible from someone who has had a stroke and offering a role model, giving them some motivation, ... I think it's been the most meaningful. That's the bit that I really treasure in a way ... what really sort of impacts on me... is giving something back and the work I do is involving stroke patients.
> (N, patient with a public sector background and member of Stroke MI Steering Group)

Service users from the stroke programme have subsequently taken a lead and ongoing role in establishing a new Stroke User Involvement Network, which sought to ensure continuity of service user engagement and support in the local area after the end of the MI programme.

Challenge 1: Defining what value the service user will add

In these consumerist times, a 'lay chair' might be considered to be a politically correct addition to any strategy or management board, but the MI discovered very early on that unless there was clarity on precisely why a service user was being appointed and what their role would be (and indeed on the role of the body they were being included on), their inclusion could be problematic. Despite a genuine commitment to user representation and input in leadership and governance, there was no user representation on the MI's highest level body, the Programme Board. There were several reasons for this. Firstly, when the Board was first set up, relations between the four trusts involved were uncertain; many stakeholders perceived that considerable risks were being taken and having service users sitting on the Board was considered yet another risk. Secondly, it was not clear at first what the role of the Board would be – to manage performance, manage the contracts or provide a forum for debate. And, without this clarity, the partners could not agree what the role or purpose of users on the Board might be. Some senior clinicians and managers subsequently reflected that user representation on the MI Board might have been beneficial, but this was not at all evident in the early days of the programme.

Our experience in the MI suggests that service users can add value in three key areas (apart from benefits to the users themselves, discussed in Challenge 5 below). First and foremost, users humanise the process of governance. Bureaucracies are in constant danger of becoming self-protecting edifices whose workers see their tasks as ends in themselves and forget the purpose for their existence. Service users act as a reminder of the people for whom the service exists, and thus as a corporate conscience. This was very powerful within the MI. Second, users in leadership and governance roles help bridge the divide between patients and professionals. As the MI progressed, there was a growth in mutual understanding and respect between the users and the professionals, with each understanding better where the other was coming from; both users and professionals gained confidence to disagree, cope with tensions, talk through problems and emerge with better solutions. And the user perspective may 'bend' projects in a more patient-centred way and serve as a lever to help push through change.

> *The chair really was our conscience, that was prickly at times, there were some frictions between me and J, between the Programme Manager and J, but that's part of it. I don't see it as being a block in any way, it was just part of the growing process. I think if you put a barrier in you stop listening and learning, you proceed as you always would, not in a new way.* (Clinical director, member of Kidney MI Steering Group)

Challenge 2: Recruiting, training and retaining users

As the two examples above show, there is no 'best formula' for recruiting users. In the Kidney MI a patient was 'hand picked' by a consultant who knew him well (the 'top down' approach); in the Stroke MI, users were recruited from join-in events advertised to all ('bottom-up'). Each initiative or service will need to be pragmatic and flexible, and anticipate that different types of users, with different skill sets and personal qualities, will be suited for particular roles in particular contexts.

In general, most users seem more interested in having direct input to service redesign than working at a more distant level. The problem of few or no applicants for a post should be anticipated, as should attrition after appointment – either because interest wanes (committee-style meetings may not be experienced as interesting or fulfilling) or because the person's condition changes or deteriorates. As the Stroke MI example above shows, effective user involvement depended on a ready supply of new service users and the infrastructure to give ongoing induction, training and support. The time commitment for front-line staff, especially the Project Managers, was greater than anticipated.

As with many 'voluntary' posts in public service, a leadership role requires considerable time commitment, flexibility and physical energy. One service user changed her job during the MI and her new work regimen gave her much less flexibility; consequently, her involvement diminished. One of the two service users appointed to the Stroke MI Steering Group stopped attending after a time because of changes in his physical condition, but he still received the papers in advance of the meetings and made his comments so they could be included in discussion. This raises an important general issue around changes in a person's health or personal circumstances during their commitment, and to what extent adjustments can or should be made to enable continued involvement (especially since the board may include people responsible for the individual's clinical care). There are no hard and fast rules here, and flexibility and sensitivity to the user's personal circumstances and the needs of the group must both be factored in.

The MI projects found that the financial and human cost of recruiting, training and retaining service users in leadership and governance roles was very significant. Costs included laying on events that users would find attractive and comfortable to attend (neutral venues, refreshments, offers of payment for attending), training users who agreed to take on leadership roles, continuing to support users who maintained a commitment, replacing users who withdrew and maintaining the 'supply chain' of new users with ongoing induction, training and support. The MI had protected funds for this work, but many public-sector bodies may struggle to find the capacity or infrastructure to undertake such work, even when all are committed to it in principle.

Challenge 3: Managing the micro-politics of the boardroom

One major challenge is ensuring that users are accepted by other members of the governance groups. Unless staff accept that the inclusion of patients and carers in a formal governance role is a good and potentially workable idea, buy-in will be low and there will not be the necessary flexibility or commitment to instigate and sustain it. The Kidney MI was perhaps unique in having a senior clinician who was known by patients and staff alike for his passion and commitment to the user perspective and his belief in this perspective to bring about transformed services. For many other staff, learning to listen to users and value their perspective took considerable time and was only partially successful (and the work of bringing staff on board was particularly onerous when staff turnover was high). Where undercurrents of dissent were present, these undoubtedly influenced the realpolitik of user involvement and required sensitive management – as the list in Box 6.3 illustrates.

Challenge 4: Supervision and performance management

Service users are not employees, but if they have formal leadership and governance roles they must be supervised and their performance evaluated and overseen in some way. Their training and development needs must be identified and planned for.

In the Kidney MI, J was appraised each year against the Chair's job description; areas for development were agreed and a plan instigated to enhance his skills. In the Stroke MI, the work of the service users was overseen in a slightly less formalised way. N's involvement leading the Living with a Disability workstream, for example, was managed by close liaison between him and the Stroke Project Manager. He was not formally appraised or subjected to the performance management procedures of the regular staff, but his input was scrutinised and he was given regular informal feedback and support. This was partly because the nature of the work was very organic and diffuse, mainly comprising building partnerships and inspiring others, so it would have been difficult to set targets or deadlines in these areas.

Significantly, whilst service users were involved in leadership and governance, and whilst they were 'managed' in some sense by paid staff in the projects, they did not themselves *manage* any staff. This meant that whilst their input was deemed important to the overall strategic direction of the projects, they could not 'dictate' particular courses of action for particular staff members or sub-projects. Nevertheless because the MI had such a strong user involvement ethos, users' recommendations were generally taken seriously by others at board and steering group level.

Challenge 5: Ensuring there is something in it for the user

As described above, the different MI projects, and different individuals within the projects, took a different approach to remuneration. Furthermore, payment did not have the same significance as it would have done in a conventional employer–employee relationship, since even those individuals who accepted a daily honorarium rate for their contribution still said they were not doing the job for the money (indeed, they did not describe it as a 'job' at all). This raises many questions about the appropriateness and level of remuneration for user input, which we discuss in Chapter 7.

The quotes from the service users in the above examples show that those who 'survive' the recruitment, selection, induction and training and succeed in making a valuable contribution to transformational leadership appear to gain a great deal both personally and (where appropriate) professionally. Knowing that you have improved services not only for yourself but also for others in a similar position is of course fulfilling in itself. We also found that many users gained knowledge that helped directly in managing their own condition and accessing and navigating the service.

Summary: Ten tips for involving users in leadership and governance

Despite some disappointments in the early stages of some projects,[11] user involvement in the MI appears to have been more successful overall compared to other programmes of similar size (see for example an initiative from Wales[12]). This is probably due at least partly to the philosophy of transformational leadership, which goes beyond a time-limited project. Transformational leadership is a whole attitude that needs to be embraced by all staff at all levels. It demands high levels of mutual trust and respect, and a willingness to put in the time and energy to remain flexible and open to innovation. Whilst the gains from this approach were felt to be substantial, they were not cheap or easy to achieve. Below, we set out some tips for those who seek to involve users in leadership and governance.

1 Service users can and often should be involved in leadership and governance, and their input may greatly help to keep strategic-level decisions focused on things that matter to patients and carers.

2 However, such involvement is very demanding in terms of time, resources and cultural change. All involved must appreciate the commitment this requires.

3 Professional staff must feel confident that they can manage the relationship, engagement and process in such a way that users' contributions are both valuable and valued. Staff training and backing from top management will help here.

4 There is no right or wrong way to find a service user to take on a leadership or governance role, what matters is finding an appropriate person for a particular role and supporting them in this role.

5 When a service user takes on a leadership role, success will be more likely when the leadership culture of the group is open, supportive and transformational.

6 When a service user takes on a project management role, absolute clarity is required including rules of engagement, deliverable targets and reimbursement.

7 Written job or role descriptions are useful for both the service user and the staff with whom they interact.

8 Contractual agreements, including remuneration, must be fully worked out to both sides' full satisfaction before user involvement begins. An honorary contract may help assure corporate governance and issues such as confidentiality.

9 Service users who become involved in projects are not necessarily 'representatives' of users in general, and should not be seen as such. Hence, having a user on a Steering Group is not a substitute for other forms of user consultation.

10 It must be remembered (where appropriate) that the service user has an illness which may compromise their ability to maintain input. Their needs as a patient must be recognised and addressed, and there may come a time when an exit route from 'user involvement' needs to be created.

References

1. Vance C, Larson E. Leadership research in business and health care. *J Nurs Sch* 2002; 3(2):165–171.
2. Ford J. Editorial to special edition on leadership. *Journal of Health Organisation and Management* 2004; 18(6):387–392.
3. Weber M. *Essays in Sociology*. Translated by H.H. Girth, C. Wright Mills. London: Routledge & Kegan Paul; 1948.
4. Alimo-Metcalfe B, Lawler J. Leadership development in UK companies at the beginning of the twenty-first century. Lessons for the NHS? *J Manag Med* 2001; 15(5):387–404.
5. Department of Health. *The NHS Plan*. London: NHS Executive; 2000.
6. Darzi A. *High Quality Health for All*. London: The Stationery Office; 2008.
7. Dawson S, Garside P, Hudson R, Bicknell C. *The Design & Establishment of the Leadership Council*. Cambridge: Judge Business School; 2009.
8. NHS Confederation. *Future Leadership; Reforming Leadership Development . . . Again*. London: NHS Confederation Publications; 2009.
9. Hasler M. *Users at the Heart. User Participation in the Governance and Operations of Social Care Regulatory Bodies*. London: Social Care Institute for Excellence; 2003.
10. Martin GP. 'Ordinary people only'; knowledge, representativeness, and the publics of public participation in healthcare. *Soc Health Illn* 2008; 30(1):35–54.
11. Fudge N, Wolfe CD, McKevitt C. Assessing the promise of user involvement in health service development: ethnographic study. *BMJ* 2008; 336(7639):313–317.
12. Adamson D, Bromiley R. *Community Empowerment in Practice. Lessons from Communities First*. York: Joseph Rowntree Foundation; 2008.

CHAPTER 7

Inherent tensions in involving users

Trisha Greenhalgh[1], *Fran Woodard*[2] *& Charlotte Humphrey*[3]
[1]Queen Mary, University of London, London, UK
[2]Integrated Cancer Centre, King's Health Partners, London, UK
[3]King's College London, London, UK

This chapter draws on the literature review (see Chapter 2) and the empirical work described in Chapters 3–6 to highlight the inherent tensions and paradoxes of trying to involve users in service transformation. The topics covered here are those we experienced in the modernisation initiative (MI), but they are probably not an exhaustive list.

Tension 1: Representation and representativeness

There is no 'view from nowhere'. In other words, everyone brings a perspective (and hence some personal interests, priorities and biases), as well as particular capabilities and limitations, to any project they are involved in. This goes for professionals too, of course, whose 'baggage' may include loyalty to their organisation and/or professional body, an interest in a particular clinical procedure or research programme, a desire to impress a senior and the world view of their own culture, religion, class and gender. Likewise, a service user may be a 'user of sexual health services' but he or she may also be rich or poor, religious or non-religious, employed or unemployed, supported by a wide network of family and friends or socially isolated, and so on. A lay member of a working group may

---

User Involvement in Health Care, 1st edition. Edited by Trisha Greenhalgh,
Charlotte Humphrey and Fran Woodard. © 2011 Blackwell Publishing Ltd.

be selected because he or she has particular knowledge or expertise in addition to being a patient or carer (e.g. experience in media, law, or committee procedure). Clearly, an individual service user does not 'represent' all others with the same disease or illness in any simple sense.

Barnes et al. have suggested three types of lay 'representativeness': (a) 'democratic' representativeness, where the individual is elected; (b) 'statistical' representativeness, where the individual is judged to be mathematically representative of a particular group (e.g. because they have neither a very mild nor a very severe form of the condition); and (c) 'typical' representativeness, where the person is considered to share key characteristics and/or experiences with the group represented (e.g. a user of dialysis services).[1]

More fundamentally, some authors have criticised the notion of considering service users (or 'the public' or 'lay people') purely in terms of their own individual characteristics. As Barnes et al. put it in a later article (p. 379):[2]

>...people may take part in participation initiatives because they have volunteered to do so or because they have been invited, exhorted or coerced. Participation may be motivated by collective experiences of oppression or exclusion, by altruistic motives associated with seeking service improvements for others or the wish to develop skills and self-confidence. The reason for participation may affect the perceived legitimacy of contributions. Different forms of participation may create different circumstances and opportunities for people to take part. [The] question of who participates cannot be answered solely by reference to individual motivation, but also needs to understand the power relations operating within any particular initiative.

The bottom line is that those who seek input from service users should eschew simplistic models of who is represented by those users, and acknowledge that like other members of steering or working groups, users bring complex identities, a range of skills and particular personal biases and limitations.

Tension 2: 'Staying naïve' or 'going native'

As Chapters 3–6 illustrate, service users often bring a fresh and sometimes naïve perspective, requiring regular staff to reconsider their assumptions, reframe their view of what the service is about, and explain and question their jargon. But the longer and more closely the user is involved in a project, the greater the risk that freshness and naïveté will be lost and that they will unconsciously take on the assumptions and world view of the staff and the organisation.

All the projects struggled with the challenge of maintaining fresh engagement of service users over time and avoiding the development of a cohort of 'usual suspects' who expected to be reinvited for every new user involvement event. On the other hand, we found that with some projects, it was impractical to keep recruiting new users and that a cohort of trained and familiar individuals brought a great deal to the initiative through their accumulated experience and familiarity with the project and with one another.

The challenge to avoid 'going native' is complicated by the fact that 'maintaining naïveté' can lead to frustration and irritation. The service user needs a certain level of understanding of the organisation and how it works in order to be effective. In the MI, for example, the ability of users to understand the programme's remit and the relationship and tensions between the MI and the participating trusts was important. The failure of some heavily involved service users to understand the relationship led, at times, to tensions that could not always be resolved in a straightforward way. A challenge for the MI Director and her staff was managing these inherent frustrations within the project.

Hogg and Williamson have suggested that when user involvement initiatives are planned, lay people tend to be defined in terms of what they are not (not professional, not knowledgeable, not socialised into organisational culture, not on the payroll and so on) rather than in terms of the positive aspects of who they are or what they might bring.[3] It is sometimes assumed (usually incorrectly) that they will therefore bring a dose of 'ordinariness' or common sense to a group otherwise composed of professionals or 'in-house' members. This of course is a naïve framing of the complex role of the 'lay member'.

In reality, Hogg and Williamson found, lay people tended to assume one of three types of interest: (a) 'dominant' interests – that is, aligning with doctors and other health professionals; (b) 'challenging' interests – that is, aligning with the executive or managerial perspective; or (c) supporting repressed [patient] interests.[3] In other words, there is no guarantee that the 'service user' on a working group will necessarily *speak for* service users – especially if they have been cajoled or coerced to join the group by a health professional and if they perceive that their leverage is weak and/or their mandate from other service users is limited.

In summary, the tension between 'staying naïve' and 'going native' is inherent, and a state of perfect naïveté combined with perfect awareness of all the relevant issues is impossible to achieve. The appropriate intensity and length of user involvement will vary according to both the task and the user(s). Ideally, users should be made aware of this tension and their help sought in addressing it.

Tension 3: Power shifts or partnerships?

In Chapter 3 we described a redesign example in which funds were spent on making a sexual health clinic 'patient-centred' with a modern, bright and welcoming physical environment, but where insufficient funds were left over for refurbishment of the staff room. In several other examples throughout the book, we allude to the need for staff input beyond what is on their job description – and occasionally time commitment for which they are not paid. These examples suggest that making the service better for users may sometimes involve a trade-off in terms of the sacrifices expected of staff.

Whilst this was occasionally the case in the MI, only a small fraction of projects could be articulated in terms of such simplistic, zero-sum ('users gain, staff lose') equations. This was partly because a user involvement initiative tended to also bring benefits for staff and the organisation. For example, the redesigned service was less stressful for staff (e.g. shorter waits for patients meant fewer complaints), staff understood their role better and felt more fulfilled and professionalised, they gained human capital in terms of qualifications or skills (and sometimes were thereby eligible for pay increments or promotion), or potential efficiency savings emerged which offered time dividends in another aspect of their work.

Arguably, framing user involvement in terms of 'shifting the power away from staff and towards users' is a politically naïve approach which will work against fundamental transformation of services. Rutter et al., for example, evaluated an initiative to involve users in improving mental health services, and concluded that because the goal of professionals had been limited to the 'empowerment' of patients in certain professionally-defined areas, the gains achieved were limited and the users' own agendas never even reached the negotiating table (p. 1973):[4]

> We found that [user involvement] remained in the gift of provider managers: providers retained control over decision making, and expected users to address Trust agendas and conform to Trust management practices. Users [also] wanted to achieve concrete changes to policies and services, but had broader aspirations to improve the status and condition of people with mental health problems.

Similar findings were produced in the evaluation of a completely different initiative in Canada, in which service users were asked in focus groups about their experiences of 'citizen participation' in healthcare policymaking.[5] They felt that whereas the policymakers viewed the focus of the project as limited to the particular policy issues chosen for discussion, their own priorities were subtly different. First, users placed greater emphasis on the content and balance of information so as to build trust and credibility between the parties. Second, users viewed themselves as sources of information (whereas policymakers tended to see their own evidence as the only valid information sources). Finally, users felt that getting the information and communication principles right was an essential precondition for (and in some ways more important than) addressing all other principles. Thus, whilst the policymakers had envisaged a simple consultation process to 'empower' the lay public in defined policymaking decisions, the lay people themselves wanted upstream negotiations on what was 'in frame' and on the nature of the lay-professional relationship.

Some research groups have explicitly moved away from an 'empowerment' model of power-sharing and sought instead to build partnerships with their service users. The partnership model does not seek to 'even out' power differentials. Rather, it acknowledges that these differentials exist and probably will always exist. The goal of the partnership model is to achieve clarity and insight on where power is located, assign responsibility, and identify and address what really matters to users (page 191):[6]

> Empowerment may be an outcome of partnership with service users, but is not its primary aim. What is important is that the users' voice is heard, their perspective is valued and their views have influence.

This resonates with our findings in the MI that staff who have little experience of involving users may feel vulnerable and anxious that they will be criticised or exposed, but once these early anxieties have been overcome the potential often develops for taking the partnership further than either side initially envisaged.

In summary, those who seek to involve users should be conscious of the tendency to define goals over-simplistically in terms of 'handing over power'. Whilst such framings may appear user-centred, productive and radical change is more likely to be achieved through partnership models.

Tension 4: To pay or not to pay users?

A recurring tension in the MI was whether and how much to pay users for their input. As previous chapters have highlighted, some staff felt strongly that users should be paid, and some but not all users accepted payment. The tension around payment or non-payment centres partly on the question of what payment is *for*, and possibilities include:

- Expenses (travel, childcare)
- Compensation for loss of earnings
- A salary for regular work
- A consultancy fee for particular specialised input
- A honorarium (i.e. a token 'thank you') for volunteering
- Payment as a signal of value: if the user is paid this conveys the message that their contribution counts and will be taken seriously

In general, it should be made clear to users that payment is not intended as a 'salary'. One high-earning service user was insulted by the amount offered for their input to a project, perhaps because this appeared to devalue the input itself. On the other hand, in the few instances where users were effectively doing a job (e.g. leading a workstream, reading and responding to committee papers), the question arose as to why the service user should not be paid the same as others who are doing the same job.

If the payment is a salary, the user effectively becomes an employee and requires line management, supervision, performance review and a stipulated notice period – all of which may help improve the quality and consistency of their input but which also fundamentally change the relationship and increase the risk of 'going native' discussed above.

Importantly, some users in the MI programme felt that whilst travel and subsistence payments were acceptable, payment for their actual input was inappropriate. They used the expression 'giving something back' to suggest that their interest and input was itself 'payment' for services received. At one extreme, users felt that they owed their lives to the service and that it was the least they could do to help improve it for the benefit of others. More generally, the public-sector ethos of the NHS engendered a strong sense of commitment and reciprocity from many of its users. It follows, perhaps, that users may feel uncomfortable if they are *required* to accept payment, and that when payment is available, accepting it should be voluntary. A further option, which we did not use in the MI but might have done, is to offer a payment to the user's chosen charity.

We found that clarity was needed not merely on how much money would be paid for input, but also on the status of the relationship. Our policy in most cases was to make explicit to users that the payment was an honorarium and did not constitute a contract of employment – and that it could be withdrawn at any time. This was relatively straightforward when the user's input was for a one-off event. When their input was expected on an ongoing basis (e.g. as a member of a steering or working group), the 'honorarium' status of the payment was more problematic – especially since considerable resources were sometimes put into training the user for the role. In a few cases (see Chapter 6), the service user was offered a consultancy fee rather than an honorarium.

When offered a payment, regardless of how much it was, the users felt that their time, input and views were being taken seriously. Many said that if the project team were bothering to pay them, this changed the accountability of the relationship significantly (users talked about 'a more serious partnership'). Payment, even at very modest levels, became an incentive for people to get involved as they felt it was worth their time (not because of the actual pay but because the pay represented that the input was valued).

Unsurprisingly, users who were financially less well off were keen on payment. Legally, if users are paid more than a certain amount, they can lose state income such as disability or unemployment benefit. Official guidance (see below) is that a small payment of up to £20 per week can be given without the individual forfeiting their regular income. Whilst cash-in-hand, on-the-day payments were undoubtedly much more acceptable to poor participants than a cumbersome system of submitting claims, such payments raised substantial governance and practical challenges (including staff safety when large amounts of cash was being handled), and in most cases we employed a formal invoicing arrangement.

Most of the MI work was undertaken before the publication of the latest Department of Health guidance on payment to service users. This guidance, *'Reward and Recognition'*, summarises the pros and cons of paying users and also places great emphasis on issues of contracting and governance, giving detail on precisely what is and is not permitted in different circumstances.[7] Another area covered in *'Reward and Recognition'* is legal restrictions on 'notional earnings' – effectively, the number of hours a volunteer who is drawing state benefits may work *without* getting paid (designed to protect volunteers from exploitation). In our experience, the use of official guidance is unlikely to put people off taking on user involvement roles. On the contrary, clarity of contract, payment and expected hours of input are essential in order for all sides to be able to work together effectively. Box 7.1 summarises the Department of Health guidance on paying service users.

Tension 5: 'First, do no harm' or 'tell it like it is'

As the examples in Chapters 3–6 show, service users' interest in participating in service transformation often stems from their personal experience, not uncommonly in relation to serious and life-threatening conditions. Whilst these experiences are often precisely what the users recruited for, they may also limit the individual's cognitive abilities, emotional stability, physical performance or stamina. Stroke patients, for example, may suffer permanent difficulty in communicating as well as emotional lability, visual impairment and mobility difficulties. People on haemodialysis need to be connected to a machine for several hours every 2–3 days, and often have anaemia and general fatigue. Those with chronic heart disease may lack energy. And so on.

The user's medical condition raises both practical and ethical issues. As our own experience (see Chapters 3–6) shows, there is a need to provide information in accessible form, modify the content and pace of meetings and ensure that all staff are fully trained in how to support users with different needs and circumstances in different involvement roles.

Box 7.1 Principles of good practice for payment and reimbursement for service user involvement (summarised from *'Reward and Recognition'*, p. 10):[7]

1 Service users should not be left out of pocket or put at risk of being financially worse off as a result of their involvement in service improvement.
2 Service providers and users should discuss and agree on the terms of involvement prior to committing to it.
3 Service users should be given the right information at the right time to be able to make an informed choice about how and on what terms they want to be involved.
4 The contribution service users make can be recognised and valued in all sorts of ways in addition to (or instead of) payment – such as being thanked, positive feedback and acknowledgement, staff time, practical assistance, training, personal development or seeing the impact of the work and changes made as a result of involvement.
5 A wide range of service users, with different needs and experiences should be encouraged and supported to be involved. The way that payment and/or reimbursement of expenses are settled should not needlessly create barriers that deter service users from being involved.
6 Service users in receipt of benefits should be provided with the right information and support to prevent a breach of their benefit conditions. Breach of benefit conditions can result in benefits being stopped.
7 Service users should be paid according to open and consistent criteria that take into account the level of involvement, the type of work and the skills and expertise required.
8 Paperwork to claim payment and reimbursement should be kept to a minimum. Where paperwork is necessary to safeguard both the service provider and the user, it should be accessible and easy to understand.

In addition, there is the question of whether it is reasonable for a patient with condition X to be exposed to discussions on the incurable nature and poor prognosis of condition X and the need (for example) to improve services for end-of-life care. In Chapter 5 we gave examples of clinicians in kidney services who perceived a widespread problem of 'denial' amongst patients, including the user representatives on working groups (though some users were very realistic about prognosis and sanguine about addressing palliative care issues in end stage kidney disease). The Kidney MI's efforts to involve users in leadership roles (see Chapter 6) also exposed users to full and frank discussions on the 'warts and all' inner workings of the NHS – including inadequate resource allocation and perceived flaws in national level policy.

Once again, there are no generalisable rules about how to handle these issues, but a core guiding principle is to consider how the issues being discussed (or which could potentially be discussed) will be framed and interpreted by the users and carers who are involved in the project. In some circumstances, users will need a debriefing session after being involved in debates and discussions.

Tension 6: 'Real' participation or 'playing the user card'?

The MI programme which forms the empirical material for this book was built on a genuine commitment to involve users in the design, delivery and evaluation of services.[8] But even in the presence of such commitment – and especially in its absence – the input of service users can come to be used instrumentally by clinicians, managers and policymakers to achieve what amounts to their own agenda. In Chapter 6, we referred to the user perspective as a 'lever for change' and in Chapter 2, we set out the policy context for user involvement and argued that, currently in the United Kingdom, the user voice is taken extremely seriously.

Back in 1998, as background to a largely theoretical paper, Harrison and Mort described an empirical study of an attempt to involve mental health service users in service redesign.[9] Whilst clinical and managerial staff espoused strongly supportive views of user involvement, they also employed strategies to dismiss or denigrate the perspective expressed (saying, for example, that the users recruited via user groups were 'not representative', poorly organised, difficult to contact or failed to care properly for their own volunteers). In this way, the professionals could draw selectively and strategically on the 'user view' (and the perception of this view as legitimate and valuable) to pursue goals they themselves deemed worthwhile.

In a more recent paper which reported an evaluation of the Better Government for Older People initiative, Williams employed the in-depth analytic technique of conversation analysis to show five different techniques used by policymakers to manage citizens' agendas and refocus the input of users around their own strategic priorities.[10]

The instrumental use of user involvement to legitimise decisions made by other stakeholders reflects the uneven power balance between users and clinicians and requires ongoing attention. The principle must surely be reflexive awareness by the project team of the existence of this danger and the use of methods (see 'partnerships' above) which minimise the risk.

Conclusion

Involving users is not easy, nor should we expect it to be. The tensions described in this chapter are inherent and therefore cannot be resolved by the use of guidelines, principles, rules or checklists. Those seeking to involve service users in any aspect of service transformation must be aware of the ambiguities and manage them on a project-by-project and situation-by-situation basis.

The bottom-line message from the different projects described in this book is that user involvement is often resource-intensive and demanding for all parties, but also that it can be a highly effective way to achieve service transformation even in settings where traditions run deep. In the next chapter, we suggest avenues for developing user involvement further, including possible research topics.

References

1. Barnes M, Harerison S, Mort M, Shardlow P. *Unequal Partners: User Groups & Community Care*. Bristol: Policy Press; 1999.
2. Barnes M, Newman J, Knops A, Sullivan H. Constituting 'the public' in public participation. *Public Adm* 2003; 81(2):379–399.
3. Hogg C, Williamson C. Whose interests do lay people represent? Towards an understanding of the role of lay people as members of committees. *Health Expect* 2001; 4(1):2–9.
4. Rutter D, Manley C, Weaver T, Crawford MJ, Fulop N. Patients or partners? Case studies of user involvement in the planning and delivery of adult mental health services in London. *Social Science & Medicine* 2004; 58(10):1973–1984.

5. Abelson J, Forest PG, Casebeer A, Mackean G. Will it make a difference if I show up and share? A citizens' perspective on improving public involvement processes for health system decision-making. *J Health Serv Res Policy* 2004; 9(4):205–212.
6. Barnes D, Carpenter J, Bailey D. Partnerships with service users in interprofessional education for community mental health: a case study. *J Interprof Care* 2000; 14(2):189–200.
7. Department of Health Care Services Improvement Partnership. *Reward and Recognition: The Principles and Practice of Service User Payment and Reimbursement in Health and Social Care*. London: Stationery Office; 2006.
8. Greenhalgh T, Humphrey C, Hughes J, Macfarlane F, Butler C, Connell P et al. *The Modernisation Initiative Independent Evaluation: Final Report*. 2008. London: University College London.
9. Harrison S, Mort M. Which champions, which people? Public and user involvement in health care as a technology of legitimation. *Soc Policy Adm* 1998; 32(1):60–70.
10. Williams M. Discursive democracy and New Labour: five ways in which decision-makers manage citizen agendas in public participation initiatives. *Sociol Res Online* 2009; 9(3): www.socresonline.org.uk/9–3/contents.html.

CHAPTER 8

Where next for user involvement?

Trisha Greenhalgh[1], Fran Woodard[2] & Charlotte Humphrey[3]
[1]Queen Mary, University of London, London, UK
[2]Integrated Cancer Centre, King's Health Partners, London, UK
[3]King's College London, London, UK

This book has described some examples, each of them to a greater or lesser extent successful, of service users being involved in transformation efforts in a programme of work that was based in the UK National Health Service but which received generous external funding from a charitable sponsor. Overall, these examples show that user involvement *can* make a significant contribution to service transformation and they highlight some approaches and caveats for making a user involvement initiative more likely to succeed.

Despite a strong and growing discourse of user involvement in policy documents (see Chapter 2 for a full literature review), the reality to date is that very few mainstream healthcare initiatives either in the United Kingdom or elsewhere have achieved the level and diversity of user involvement needed to have a major impact on transforming services. This is partly because such involvement would probably require costly pump-priming investment as well as an ongoing budget line, but it is also because the substantial cultural changes required for user involvement to become 'business as usual' in public-sector healthcare are yet to occur.

Currently, much user involvement in healthcare is limited to 'special projects' – either led by a particular champion or funded from a particular short-term resource. We are still a long way from

User Involvement in Health Care, 1st edition. Edited by Trisha Greenhalgh, Charlotte Humphrey and Fran Woodard. © 2011 Blackwell Publishing Ltd.

the situation depicted in some policy documents where users are *routinely* involved in all aspects of the service and their involvement is a 'non-issue' for both staff and the users themselves (in the same way, perhaps, that the Guardian newspaper abolished its 'women's page' several years ago on the grounds that the issues it covered had become mainstream ones for all readers).

One question for policymakers and planners is 'What would user involvement look like once it has become business as usual?' Below, we consider some radical possibilities and outline areas for future research. These suggestions are deliberately speculative and intended to open up debate rather than as a definitive agenda.

Abolishing 'user involvement' bodies – or developing their role?

If user involvement were successfully mainstreamed, it could obviate the need for the various specialist agencies that have waxed and waned over the years such as Community Health Councils, Patient Advice and Liaison Service and Local Involvement Networks (see Chapter 2). Indeed, it could be argued that the mainstream embedding of user involvement across all aspects of the service would *require* the abolition of these special agencies as their different roles and linkages were built more centrally and holistically into the service.

On the other hand, given the intrinsic power differentials and mismatch of priorities between patients and professionals, the idea that the user voice could ever be mainstreamed without conflict (or at least, negotiation) seems implausible. A research agenda on user involvement bodies could consider (for example) how such bodies might interface more effectively with transformational initiatives in health services and how new forms of partnership could generate inspiration and energy for making and sustaining changes to services.

User networks

One way of going beyond a situation where a service has a cohort of 'usual suspects' – users upon whom they call for input when this is deemed necessary – is to encourage the development of a *network* of users. The remit of such a network might include providing a point of access for services seeking user input, helping to recruit, train and support volunteers, matching particular users to particular projects, spreading the workload among volunteers, encouraging new users to take part, and stimulating user-led initiatives.[1]

In some MI projects, the combination of a strong user involvement ethos and a critical mass of involved users meant that some users spontaneously began to take responsibility for ensuring breadth and diversity of input. For example, established users in one project sometimes took on the task of recruiting new participants to the project, and others moved on from taking a 'seasoned' role in one initiative to being a relatively naïve member of another project. In other words, a 'network' model seems to promote flexible and changing involvement rather than entrenchment of roles.

User networking was the subject of a report by the Joseph Rowntree Foundation.[2] Whilst the ability to network is greatly valued by users who participate, it is not easy to organise. Problems identified in this report included limitations of mobility and commitment by users, the fragility of user-controlled organisations, inadequate and insecure funding and limited facility to engage 'harder to reach' users (e.g. limited English speakers) in the network because of lack of funding. Our own experience suggests that – unsurprisingly – users tend to get involved most readily with issues that interest and concern them and are much less willing to be involved in things they either do not understand or cannot see the relevance of. There is a research agenda here to identify what works for whom in what circumstances in relation to user networks and to explore how user interest and engagement might be matched with available roles for involvement.

Promises and pitfalls of new technologies

Internet technologies are sometimes hailed as a particularly effective way of communicating with users and capturing the user perspective (see, for example, the UK government's 'e-government' website on http://archive.cabinetoffice.gov.uk/e-government/).[3] Linking with users in this way may be seen as 'democratising' and therefore liberating – but as Michel Foucault and others after him have pointed out, such technologies also greatly increase the potential for state surveillance and control of citizens. Foucault appropriated the term 'panopticon' from the liberal philosopher Jeremy Bentham to highlight how the state has ever-increasing power to scrutinise our professional and private lives without us being consciously aware of this.[4] Even when we are being 'consulted' in an e-government initiative, the state is able to build into the technology the range of issues on which consultation will happen and the range of possible responses to closed questions (e.g. via a pull-down menu).

When we were evaluating the user involvement work of the MI, we were struck by the preponderance of personal, low technology approaches such as small-scale face-to-face meetings or phone calls from a known and trusted nurse. Whilst contemporary rhetoric on achieving 'democratic' user involvement via new technologies is strong, in reality such involvement may be highly institutionalised and constrained by the assumptions and discourses that have been deliberately or inadvertently built into the technologies as symbols, data models and decision paths. As Richter et al have put it:

> *Of particular interest is the notion of the e-Citizen, set against a contemporary public management backdrop featuring customer-centric discourses/metaphors, organisational transformation and ICT-intensive 'private-sector' business solutions* (p. 207).[5]

More prosaically, high-tech consultation initiatives are often limited by practical and technical issues. As one group of researchers put it:

> *[e-government] is often thwarted by a host of intricacies contributed by the lack of ICT resources and infrastructure, unequal access to technology, low e-literacy rate and the lack of appropriate government policy initiatives and commitments* (p. 156).[6]

Clearly, whilst there is great theoretical potential for achieving user involvement 'via the Internet', there are many unanswered research questions in relation to the various social, political, economic and technical barriers to this goal.

The role of the third sector

Because they were based largely within the NHS and delivered by temporarily redeployed NHS staff, the projects described in this book were essentially public-sector initiatives. Voluntary sector organisations were invited to become involved in different ways (for example, they were consulted in relation to what the MI's priorities should be and offered representation on its various management and governance structures). These linkages were often (though perhaps not always) very fruitful and allowed the user voice to be conveyed 'indirectly' via an organisation such as the Terrence Higgins Trust (HIV), the Kidney Patients Association or Connect (people living with stroke).

Other models of user involvement, in which changes in public-sector services are initiated, driven and evaluated by the third sector, were beyond the scope of this book. But there is a small and important additional literature describing potential models for such input – ranging from formal and amicable partnerships with the public sector to critical (and sometimes confrontational) challenges to the prevailing service models.[7–11] User involvement projects often need to balance the conflicting relationships between voluntary and statutory organisations and with the users themselves. Voluntary organisations have played a key role in social movements in the United States and United Kingdom, particularly with mental health service users,[7] and have long been proponents of involving service users in the education and training of health professionals and service providers. There is scope for much more research in this area.

The link between self-management and user involvement in service transformation

In parallel with the prevailing rhetoric on user involvement in change and quality improvement, another discourse on self-management of illness often appears in the same policy documents.[12–15] Self-management (via initiatives such as the expert patient – see Chapter 2) is seen by many policymakers as both empowering for patients and potentially cost-saving for the health service. However, critics have suggested that 'expert patient' programmes, like user involvement initiatives, have a strong political dimension and are not necessarily as empowering as the name implies.[16, 17]

One of our findings in the evaluation of the MI was that neither self-care nor user involvement saved time, nor did they generate significant cost savings for the service in the short term – mainly because both required an infrastructure (for registration, training, support and so on) to sustain them. Furthermore, we did not find an especially strong link between the desire and ability to play an active role in managing one's own chronic illness and the desire to help [re]design services.

User involvement in the design of services could potentially produce medium-term savings in some areas (for example, if sexual health services were more accessible and popular with users, the prevalence of sexually transmitted diseases and the number of unwanted pregnancies locally could be reduced); however, it would be difficult (though perhaps not impossible) to demonstrate that such indirect benefits were 'caused' by a particular user involvement initiative. Again, the costs and cost-effectiveness of user involvement and the links between promoting self-management and engaging users in service transformation are largely speculative and further research to elucidate these links would be welcome – especially at a time when the costs of healthcare are rising and the budget for providing it is falling rapidly in real terms.

Towards more sophisticated evaluation of user involvement

Traditionally, a programme was said to have worked if the goal(s) originally set out by its designers were achieved on time and within budget. 'Evaluation' was conflated with audit or accounting and consisted of largely quantitative data which could answer questions of the general format 'how much...?', 'how quickly...?' or 'what proportion of...?'. The science of evaluation has advanced considerably in recent years, and where complex policy interventions are concerned there is increasing emphasis on qualitative and mixed-methods research which seeks to determine not merely *whether* an initiative was successful but how and in what ways it was successful – or, alternatively, to find plausible explanations for its 'failure'.[18–21]

Indeed, it has been argued that the very notions of 'success' and 'failure' are socially constructed (i.e. in the eye of the beholder), and a key first task for the evaluator is to ascertain what different stakeholders in the project view as 'success' and under what circumstances they consider that it would have 'failed'.[22]

Our evaluation of the various MI projects described in this book was informed by three closely related approaches. The first was Utilisation-Focused Evaluation, developed by Professor Michael Quinn Patton.[19] This approach has parallels with what Paul Bate once described as 'studying quality qualitatively'.[23] Patton defined programme evaluation as '*the systematic collection of information about the characteristics, activities and outcomes of programs to make judgements about the program, improve program effectiveness, and/or inform decisions about future programming'* [p. 33].

In other words, utilisation focused evaluation seeks to generate data and interpretations which policymakers and other stakeholders can make practical use of (for example, to modify particular goals or efforts as the project unfolds). Secondly, we were inspired by John Ovretveit's 'action evaluation' approach, in which what is essentially a utilisation-focused approach is combined with a more explicit action research methodology to actively inform and help drive changes to services.[24]

The third approach which informed our evaluation of the MI user involvement work was realist evaluation, developed by Pawson and Tilley.[21] Realist evaluation asks the question 'what works for whom in what circumstances?' in studying the dynamic relationship between context, mechanism and outcome (sometimes referred to using the shorthand term 'C-M-O'). Both realist and utilisation-focused evaluation recognise that a complex programme of work tends to unfold in unpredictable ways and that goals and milestones are (sometimes very appropriately) renegotiated along the way – hence an experimental approach (e.g. a randomised controlled trial) may be a less appropriate study design than one which aims to build a rich picture of a story unfolding over time.[25, 26] Realist evaluation is especially interested in theories of change – that is, in the *mechanisms by which* particular outcomes might be achieved, given the right contextual conditions.[27–29]

The principles of realist evaluation can also be used to synthesise findings from more than one evaluation study (a technique known as realist review, involving a systematic search for C-M-O configurations across multiple primary studies).[30] Daykin et al. undertook a realist review of a sample of eight different user involvement initiatives in healthcare and concluded that three key domains help determine outcome.[31] These were: (a) structure and resources (i.e. organisational structures that support partnership working, programme-level structures to support staff and safeguard users, and mechanisms to measure impact); (b) politics and discourse (for example, they comment that 'consumerist models of engagement and bureaucratic forms of consultation were widely reported as alienating for lay participants' [p. 59], but that models of discursive democracy and community development tended to increase users' ability to influence outcomes); and (c) attitudes and culture (the extent to which professionals were threatened by, and/or accepting of, users at the front line of efforts to change services).

A full exploration of the merits and challenges of realist and other 'mostly qualitative' approaches to evaluation is beyond the scope of this book (though we have considered this question in relation to the MI in a published paper and internal report[32, 33]).

Interested readers might also like to visit the website of the User Involvement in Voluntary Organisations Shared Learning Group (http://www.user-involvement.org.uk/) which offers some downloadable documents offering practical advice on how to evaluate a user involvement initiative. These authors rightly emphasise the subtle and non-linear nature of user impact (and hence the high chance that an experimental, quantitative approach to evaluation risks missing important findings). For example, they cite a health professional who commented that '*I spoke to a user who made me think about the issue differently, which meant that in the next meeting I argued the case in a way that I don't normally do, which made someone else get angry and argue their point more passionately which then persuaded the others to do something different... How do you describe that impact? You may have to experience user involvement before you can fully appreciate the difference that it makes*' (p. 3).[34]

In sum, whilst we would all probably readily agree that a user involvement initiative needs to be evaluated, the detail of how best to go about this almost always requires careful consideration. Rigorous research into the methodology of evaluation in these complex change initiatives would undoubtedly add to the knowledge base.

Conclusion

We know that involving service users in change efforts can be effective in various ways, but we also know that is difficult, demanding and has significant resource implications. But as the ideas, reports and preliminary studies outlined in this chapter show, there is much we still do not know about user involvement in service transformation initiatives. At this time when NHS resources are being reduced in real time, it may be unrealistic to expect research and development in the field of user involvement work to be funded entirely from within the NHS. We suggest it is time to consider imaginative partnerships between the NHS, academia and the third sector to take forward this potentially far-reaching agenda.

References

1. Tew J, Gell C, Foster S. *Learning From Experience: Involving Service Users and Carers in Mental Health Education and Training. Mental Health in Higher Education.* National Institute for Mental Health in England (West Midlands). Nottingham: Trent Workforce Development Confederation; 2004.

2. Branfield F, Beresford P. *Making User Involvement Work: Supporting User Networking and Knowledge.* York: Joseph Rowntree Foundation; 2006.

3. Palvia SCJ, Sharma SS. *E-Government and E-Governance: Definitions/Domain Framework and Status around the World.* 2007. Downloadable from http://www.iceg.net/2007/books/1/1_369.pdf. International Congress on e-Government.

4. Foucault M. *Discipline and Punish: The Birth of the Prison.* New York: Random House; 1975.

5. Richter P, Cornford J, McLoughlin I. The e-Citizen as talk, as text and as technology: CRM and e-Government. *Electron J e-Gov* 2004; 2(3):207–218.

6. As-Saber S, Hossain K, Srivastava A. Technology, society and e-government: in search of an eclectic framework. *Electr Gov – Int J* 2007; 4(2):156–178.

7. Bate SP, Robert G, Bevan H. Mobilising for the next phase of NHS modernisation: building a movement. *Qual Saf Health Care* 2004; 13(1):62–66.

8. Doyal L. Changing medicine? Gender and the politics of health care. In: Gabe D, Kelleher D, editors. *Challenging Medicine.* London: Routledge; 1994.

9. Kelleher D. Self-help groups and their relationship to medicine. In: Gabe J, Kelleher D, Williams G, editors. *Challenging Medicine.* London: Routledge; 1994.

10. Levy JM, Storeng KT. Living positively: Narrative strategies of living with HIV in Cape Town, South Africa. *Anthropol Med* 2007; 14(1):55–68.

11. Donaldson A, Lank E. Connecting through communities: how a voluntary organization is influencing healthcare policy and practice. *J Change Manage* 2005; 5(1):71–86.

12. Department of Health. *Self Care – A Real Choice.* London: Department of Health; 2005.

13. Department of Health. *Our Health, Our Care, Our Say: A New Direction for Community Services.* London: The Stationery Office; 2006.

14. Department of Health. *Putting People First: A Shared Vision and Commitment to the Transformation of Adult Social Care.* London: The Stationery Office; 2007.

15. Darzi A. *High Quality Health for All*. London: The Stationery Office; 2008.
16. Osborne RH, Jordan JE, Rogers A. A critical look at the role of self-management for people with arthritis and other chronic diseases. *Nat Clin Pract Rheumatol* 2008; 4(5):224–225.
17. Clarke J. New Labour's citizens: activated, empowered, responsibilized, abandoned? *Crit Soc Policy* 2005; 25(4):447–463.
18. Guba E, Lincoln Y. *Fourth Generation Evaluation*. London: Sage; 1989.
19. Patton MQ. *Utilization-focused Evaluation: The New Century*, (3rd edition). London: Sage; 1997.
20. Potvin L, Haddad S, Frohlich KL. Beyond process and outcome evaluation: a comprehensive approach for evaluating health promotion programmes. *WHO Reg Publ Eur Ser* 2001; (92):45–62.
21. Pawson R, Tilley N. *Realistic Evaluation*. London: Sage; 1997.
22. Klecun E, Cornford T. A critical approach to evaluation. *Eur J Inf Syst* 2005; 14:229–243.
23. Bate SP, Robert G. Studying health care 'quality' qualitatively: the dilemmas and tensions between different forms of evaluation research within the UK National Health Service. *Qual Health Res* 2002; 12(7):966–981.
24. Øvretveit J. *Action Evaluation of Health Programmes and Changes. A Handbook for a User-focused Approach*. Oxford: Radcliffe; 2002.
25. Berwick DM. The science of improvement. *JAMA* 2008; 299(10):1182–1184.
26. Barnes M, Matka E, Sullivan H. Evidence, understanding and complexity: evaluation in non-linear systems. *Evaluation* 2003; 9(3):265–284.
27. Byng R, Norman I, Redfern S. Using realistic evaluation to evaluate a practice-level intervention to improve primary healthcare for patients with long-term mental illness. *Evaluation* 2005; 11(1):69–93.
28. Connell P, Kubisch AC. Applying a theory of change approach to the evaluation of comprehensive community initiatives: progress, prospects and problems. In: Fulbright-Anderson K, Kubisch AC, Connell P, editors. *New Approaches to Evaluating Community Initiatives: Vol 2. Theory, Measurement and Analysis*. Washington: Aspen Institute; 1998.
29. Pedersen LH, Rieper O. Is realist evaluation a realistic approach for complex reforms? *Evaluation* 2008; 14(3):271–293.
30. Pawson R, Greenhalgh T, Harvey G, Walshe K. Realist review–a new method of systematic review designed for complex policy interventions. *J Health Serv Res Policy* 2005; 10 Suppl 1:21–34.
31. Daykin N, Evans D, Petsoulas C, Sayers A. Evaluating the impact of patient and public involvement initiatives on UK health services: a systematic review. *Evidence and Policy* 2007; 3(1):47–65.
32. Greenhalgh T, Humphrey C, Hughes J, Macfarlane F, Butler C, Connell P et al. *The Modernisation Initiative Independent Evaluation: Final*

Report. 2008. London: University College London (downloadable from http://www.ucl.ac.uk/openlearning/research.htm).

33. Greenhalgh T, Humphrey C, Hughes J, Macfarlane F, Butler C, Pawson R. How do you modernize a health service? A realist evaluation of whole-scale transformation in London. *Milbank Q* 2009; 87(2): 391–416.

34. Anonymous. *Evaluating User Involvement*. Document 90. London: User Involvement in Voluntary Organisations Shared Learning Group; 2008. Downloadable from http://www.user-involvement.org.uk.

Index